MARK

MARK

How a Boy's Courage in Facing AIDS
Inspired a Town and the Town's Compassion
Lit Up a Nation

JAY HOYLE

Langford Books
an imprint of
Diamond Communications, Inc.
South Bend, Indiana

1988

MARK
Copyright © 1988 by Langford Books,
an imprint of Diamond Communications, Inc.

Manufactured in the United States of America

LANGFORD BOOKS/DIAMOND COMMUNICATIONS, INC.
POST OFFICE BOX 88
SOUTH BEND, INDIANA 46624
(219) 287-5008

LIBRARY OF CONGRESS
Library of Congress Cataloging-in-Publication Data

Hoyle, Jay, 1947–
    Mark : how a boy's courage in facing AIDS inspired a
town and the town's compassion lit up a nation / Jay Hoyle.
        p.   cm.
    ISBN 0–912083–30–1 : $18.95
    1. Hoyle, Mark, 1972–1986 — Health.   2. AIDS
(Disease) — Patients — Massachusetts — Biography.   I. Title.
RC607.A26H69   1988
362.1'9892'97920 — dc19   88–15466
[B]   CIP

Acknowledgments

Many who touched our lives during Mark's illness are not mentioned in this book. Some are doctors, nurses, and hospital personnel. Others are neighbors, teachers, co-workers, students, acquaintances, and friends. My family and I want them to know that we have not forgotten any of them, nor shall we ever forget what they did.

I would like to thank my publisher, Jill Langford, president of Diamond Communications, for her understanding, guidance, and willingness to give me the opportunity to tell Mark's story. To Ann Pouk, also of Diamond, I would like to extend my sincere appreciation for her cheerful enthusiasm and assistance.

Finally, and most importantly, special thanks to my wife Dale and son Scott. Without their love and encouragement, I never would have completed this endeavor.

Publisher's Note

In the course of my work on the promotion of **MARK**, an editor of a national magazine asked me to prove how the story of Mark Hoyle differs from countless other stories about AIDS victims. With the AIDS crisis in the headlines daily, I can understand his need to know what is so special about **MARK.** After all, **MARK** does resemble those stories, in that it too tells of the same devastation of the disease and the reality of death. Yet, at the same time, this book at once addresses and resolves a crucial issue of human rights. Moreover, it steps beyond the dire headlines and clinical statistics to bring to light an account that is both an inspiration and a reaffirmation of basic human goodness in the face of emotional and physical crises. This is clearly evident in the character of a boy . . . a family . . . and a community. . . .

Although physically weakened by the dual diseases of hemophilia and AIDS, Mark exhibited an emotional strength and bravery uncharacteristic of one his age . . . or any age. Without a doubt, Mark's strength of character was nurtured by a unique family foundation. In the midst of the disintegration of traditional family life, the closeness of the Hoyles defies this trend in a most heartwarming and affirming way.

Not enough can be said about the community of Swansea, Massachusetts, where the Hoyle family struggle was rooted. This small town will be hailed and honored for its steadfastness and for the bold precedent it set in support of Mark and his family. Perhaps most moving was the demonstration by the children of Swansea of their simple, unconditional love for their stricken friend and classmate.

In order to make this book as informative and educational as possible, we have elected to include, almost in its entirety, the proceedings of the meeting for parents of students at Joseph

Case Junior High School. It was here that their fears and concerns about AIDS were addressed by educators and medical personnel, and it was precisely this openness to discussion that allowed Swansea residents to react to Mark's illness with compassion rather than with hysteria. By including this meeting in Chapter 3, we hope that we are providing a model for future debate of this kind which, undoubtedly and unfortunately, will have to take place in other cities and which *should* have taken place in locations such as Kokomo, New York City, and DeSoto County, Florida.

We would like to extend very special thanks to Joyce Chatfield of Attleboro, Massachusetts; out of true friendship and concern, she first brought the Hoyle story to our attention in 1985. Additionally, we would like to thank the following for their enthusiastic cooperation and assistance in this project: Chris Callis and Karen Hadan of Chris Callis Studios in New York; Edward Durand, *Fall River Herald-News*; Rev. James M. Fitzpatrick, St. John the Evangelist Church; Mark Patinkin, *Providence Journal-Bulletin*; Bernie Sullivan, formerly with the *Providence Journal-Bulletin*, now with the *Fall River Herald-News*; and to the regional newspapers which assisted us in providing photographs, for which proper credit is given within the photographic section of this book.

And, finally, we would like to express to Dale, Jay, and Scott Hoyle how very proud we are that **MARK** is the first title of our new imprint, Langford Books. Although we know this book cannot fill the great void in your lives, we do hope that it will stand in soothing tribute to the most treasured spirit of Mark Gardiner Hoyle. Until the headlines herald a cure for AIDS, we must look to stories such as yours for our hope and resolve.

Jill A. Langford

This book is dedicated in memory of a very special young man, Mark Gardiner Hoyle. His friendly smile and gentle personality will never be forgotten by those who knew him best. Mark seemed to bring out the best in people. He was an innocent victim who created many heroes. Doctors, school administrators, teachers, students, and Swansea townspeople all rallied around him. This tremendous encouragement and support from so many individuals was deeply appreciated by Mark. To me, Mark is the real hero, he taught us all to remember, "A winner never quits and a quitter never wins; it's never too late to rally."

1

"You should just enjoy life as you can."

—Mark Hoyle

The Giants were winning six to two. Our son Mark, age 12, had pitched three good innings, striking out four, walking just one, and giving up only three singles. The two runs were unearned. But Mark said he wasn't feeling well and couldn't go on. Scott, our younger son, age 10, replaced him and Mark left the dugout to sit in the car with his mother. I was a coach and scorekeeper at the time. We eventually lost the game, 10–7, when the Dodgers came up with six runs in the bottom of the fifth. The date was Wednesday, May 22, 1985, and it was the first indication that something wasn't quite right with Mark.

Mark had joined the Swansea, Massachusetts, Little League when he was eight years old. In his first season he won the David Reynolds Memorial Trophy honoring the "most enthusiastic player." He had natural talent and considering his handicaps, he was an excellent ballplayer. Mark had severe hemophilia, but you would have never known it by looking at him. His ankles and right elbow had been major problem areas, but he always played like he was the healthiest kid around. He had to receive a needle before each game or practice. Putting the needle into a vein is not the easiest task in the world, but Mark learned how to give it to himself. He wanted to be able to care for himself and he did.

Hemophilia is a disease that people have heard about, but one about which most know very little. It is a hereditary disorder of blood clotting. The hemophiliac does not produce one of the plasma proteins needed to form a clot. The protein lacking is called antihemophilic factor, or AHF, or factor VIII. When a hemophiliac is injured, he does not bleed harder or faster than normal, but the bleeding does not stop because the hemo-

1

philiac can't make a firm clot to plug the torn blood vessels. The most common variety of hemophilia is called hemophilia A, or classical hemophilia, and this is what both Mark and Scott had. There are also three classifications of hemophiliacs: severe, moderately severe, and mild. Both Mark and Scott were classified as severe; Mark with less than 1% clotting, Scott with 4%.

Hemophiliacs sometimes require prophylactic treatments in which factor VIII is injected on a regular basis before a possible injury or bleed occurs. Usually these precautionary treatments are done daily or every other day. Although hemophilia can be treated with injections of factor VIII, there is no cure for the disorder nor prevention of the painful consequences it causes. Repeated bleeding into the joints of the hemophiliac eventually causes a type of arthritis. Mark had arthritis in both ankles and his right elbow. The repeated bleeds into his right elbow caused him to have an arm that would not go straight. Even so he was able to play baseball and play it well.

On Thursday, May 23, we took Mark to our pediatrician's office. We usually saw Dr. Roger Lemaire, but he wasn't on duty that night and we saw Dr. Jack Delaney. The doctor thought that Mark probably had some mild infection and that he would be feeling better in a day or so. It was nothing to worry about.

The week went on and Mark seemed better. The next game for the Giants was Monday, May 27, Memorial Day. Mark said he was well enough to play. It was Brian Mello's turn to pitch and Mark played shortstop. He did well in the field, but you could tell he wasn't up to par because he struck out three times, not a normal performance for a boy who had been an All-Star since age eight. After the game, Mark said he didn't feel well and we decided to take him to a walk-in clinic in Swansea. We had never been there before, but we wanted a second opinion. The doctor did not think anything was serious either, probably just a virus. We went home relieved that the two doctors had agreed.

Two days later we had another game, but Mark was too sick to play. He was back at shortstop for the next game on June 3. He went one for three with a walk and seemed much more healthy. But when he ran around the bases making a triple, he seemed more out of breath than usual. Reggie Desnoyers, the manager, asked Mark if he wanted to be taken out of the game, but he waved that he was "OK" and stayed in.

The next night we were back at the Little League complex. Mark said he felt all right and he pitched the last three innings. He went one for three again at bat and gave up just one run over the three innings. He struck out three Yankee batters. This would be his last game for a few months.

When we got home, Mark lay down on the patio glider and told us that he just hadn't been feeling well lately. His appetite wasn't as good as usual either.

We made an appointment at Fall River Pediatrics again. This time we did see Dr. Lemaire, who reassured us that it was probably just a stubborn virus, and he would get better in time. The date was June 5.

As each day went on, Mark became weaker. He missed a lot of school. He was in the seventh grade at Case Junior High School and was an honor roll student. He loved school and worked very hard to keep his grades up. Back in March, he had won second place in the Science Fair doing his project on "Hemophilia." He went to the Southeast Regional Science Fair which was held at Bristol Community College in Fall River, Massachusetts. He won third place and was very pleased. His project was a study of whether he would have more or fewer bleeds coming off prophylactic treatment. He had been receiving his factor VIII every other day for years, and he wanted to get it only when he needed it.

Mark's health continued to worsen. I called every day from work to see how he was doing. My wife, Dale, never had any good news for me. Here I was teaching healthy junior high children every day, and there was my own junior high child getting sicker and sicker. Soon he couldn't even walk to the bathroom without help. Dale and I were getting extremely worried. We had gone to three different doctors, he had been given medications, but instead of getting better, he got worse.

June 6 was graduation at my school. It was my 16th year teaching at St. John the Evangelist School in Attleboro, Massachusetts. I love teaching and I love the kids, but this year I found it hard to concentrate on the ceremony. As I read the names of the graduates from the podium at St. John Church, my mind was really on Mark. After the ceremony, I excused myself, and hurried back to Swansea, a distance of about 18 miles.

Mark had missed me and was happy to see me. We had a very special relationship. Not only was I Mark's father, I was his best friend. I felt so sorry for him; he seemed to be so weak, and I was helpless to do anything to make him better. He gave me a big hug, as only Mark could do, and I was pleased that he still could squeeze me so tightly. Scott was a big help during all this. He waited on his brother and got him anything he needed. We were a very close family; we always did everything together. The four of us could face any problems that life could present because we had each other to lean on.

Mark continued to get sicker and sicker. The weekend passed and I called my principal, Sister Martha Mulligan, R.S.M., and told her I wouldn't be able to teach that day. It was Monday, June 10, and although my eighth grade class had graduated, I still had my other history classes to teach—grades 5, 6, and 7. But I just couldn't go to school, I had to take Mark to our pediatrician again. Something more than a virus was attacking him and we had to find help for him.

When we arrived, Mark was so weak that I carried him in. Dr. Lemaire was on duty and it soon became obvious to him that Mark needed to be admitted to the hospital. One of the nurses went across the street to the hospital, St. Anne's, and brought back a wheelchair. I pushed him across to the hospital and he was admitted to the Pediatric Wing.

Mark was immediately put into intensive care. The nurse took his case history, and he was ready to be seen by the doctors. Two residents from Boston Floating were on duty that month. They were both nice, but seemed very young. They examined him, not giving any indication of what they thought was wrong. Even though Mark was obviously in poor health, he could breathe all right and didn't need oxygen then. But he couldn't get out of bed to stand. He was so terribly weak. The doctors said it could be pneumonia, TB, or a virus. Much later, we found out that AIDS, acquired immune deficiency syndrome, was put down as a possibility. His earlier X-rays didn't show much, and his white count wasn't high, so it didn't look like an infection.

Meanwhile, my sister, Jayne Wilson, had talked about Mark to Dr. Nick Mucciardi, a pulmonary expert. Jayne worked in the X-ray department at Charlton Memorial Hospital in Fall River. She explained to him about Mark and he offered to be a consultant in the case. He came that night to talk to Mark, Dale, and me. Scott was left at his grandmother's house—Nana Fazzina, as we call her.

After looking at the X-rays, Dr. Mucciardi determined that Mark had pneumonia. He wanted to do a bronchoscopy to determine what kind of pneumonia he had. We consented and he explained the procedure to Mark. Mark would be drugged into a relaxed state, and then a tube would be inserted down his throat and into his lungs. A washing from Mark's lungs would be suctioned up. This material would be tested to determine exactly what kind of pneumonia was present.

Dr. Mucciardi was a very pleasant, easy going person. He had come from the famed Lahey Clinic near Boston and, as it turned out, was also my father's doctor (Papa Hoyle as the kids called him). Mark seemed to like him right away and put his trust in him. Later Dr. Lemaire came over and also explained everything they planned to do. He was also a very likeable man. He had been Mark's principal pediatrician since birth.

Being in the hospital didn't seem to bother Mark. In fact, I think he felt a lot better there knowing that he was getting the proper care. The nurses were all nice and they gave him a great deal of attention since he was in the intensive care unit.

We promised Mark that one of us would stay with him every night until we could take him home again. This started the tradition that we followed through all of his subsequent hospital stays. Although other relatives offered to relieve us, he preferred to have one of us there, and we didn't let him down. Dale stayed the first night, and then we usually alternated nights all through his stay. Whoever went home would spend time with Scott at night. In the mornings we would get him to his Grandmother Fazzina's house so he could get the school bus. Then we would relieve each other so that the one who had been with Mark could go home and take a shower. Meanwhile, Scott would stay with Grandmother Hoyle or Fazzina after school until one of us came home to him. It was very hard on Scott, but he understood and made cards for his brother. The two brothers communicated via tape recordings like the close friends they were.

Tuesday morning, June 11, the day of the bronchoscopy, I arrived early with the factor VIII from home and gave Mark the required dose. Dr. Mucciardi had talked to our hematologist in Providence, Rhode Island, Dr. Peter Smith. They would keep in close contact throughout Mark's stay. The time arrived, and we went on the elevator with Mark to the operating room. We kissed him good-bye and wished him good luck. They wheeled his bed through the swinging doors and he was gone. It was a beautiful, warm, sunny day, and it reminded me of the day when Mark was born.

Mark Gardiner Hoyle was born on August 2, 1972. It was one of the happiest days of my life. My wife had had two miscarriages, caused by fibroid tumors, but this time her pregnancy would go the full nine months. By Caesarian section, a beautiful 7 lb. 13 oz. boy was born into this world. Everyone had thought we were going to have a girl. All our relatives and friends kept saying they could tell by the way Dale was carrying. They had me so convinced that when I went to the hospital that morning, I wore a pink shirt. It was kind of different getting up that August morning and knowing for sure that I was going to be a daddy that day. I arrived in the waiting room about 8:15 A.M. or so and I didn't have too long to wait when they told me it was a boy! I just couldn't believe it! I mean I would have loved to have had a girl, but a first born son is really something special to a father. My wife was fine, the baby seemed healthy, and I couldn't have been happier.

But a couple of days later, bad news set in. When we had Mark circumcised, he didn't stop bleeding. His blood counts went very low and he had to be transferred to Boston Floating Hospital. My parents drove me up to Boston. My mother held the baby. Dale was still at Truesdale Hospital recovering from her "section." We had never been to Boston Floating before and all the parking lots were full. My father found a place in a No Parking zone. Of course, with our luck, he got a ticket.

They shaved Mark's beautiful dark hair and put an IV needle into his head so they could give him a blood transfusion. He spent two weeks there before we could take him home. It was then that we found out he had hemophilia. It was a complete shock to both of us. By necessity we had to learn what we could about the disorder. We found out that only a woman can carry the defective gene and only males can contract hemophilia. One out of every 10,000 males born will have hemophilia. A woman is called a carrier of hemophilia if she has an abnormal gene for factor VIII or factor IX, a hemophilia gene, on the x-chromosome, which she received from one parent, and a normal gene for the factor on the x-chromosome from the other parent. The effects of the hemophilia gene are covered up by the normal gene so that she will generally not show symptoms of the disease. She can, however, pass the hemophilia gene on to her children. A male has only one x-chromosome. The y-chromosome is different and does not contain many of the genes found on the x-chromosome. It does not have genes for the production of factor VIII or factor IX. Thus, if a male inherits an x-chromosome carrying the hemophilia gene, he will show the disease because there is no normal gene on the y-chromosome to cover up the effects of the hemophilia gene. In other words, we had a 50/50 chance (but didn't know it) that if we had a girl she would be a carrier, and a 50/50 chance, that if we had a boy, he would have hemophilia.

The bronchoscopy went well. Dr. Mucciardi told us that Mark fought it a little, so they gave him a little more medication and he was able to get it down with no problem. We had thought Mark would be completely unconscious when the procedure was done and we felt bad for him—especially me, because I can't even swallow an aspirin! I could just imagine the awful feeling of having a tube put down my throat.

Mark came back to the room and then had a severe bout of the chills. He was freezing and we couldn't do anything to ease his shaking. The nurses brought extra blankets and I climbed into the bed with him to warm him. It was just terrible! His teeth were chattering and everything. But after about 30 minutes of this, he calmed down and was better.

His throat was very dry and he was extremely thirsty, but he didn't complain. He always had the philosophy: "A winner never quits, and a quitter never wins." He was a positive thinker. "It's never too late to rally," he would say and he meant it.

He loved to win and he always played every game with that

intention. I had taught him how to play checkers when he was young and before long he was beating me. He learned how to play chess in grammar school and got many tips from his Uncle Dale (my sister's husband). Before long he was beating everyone at that too. In fact, when Mark was in grade six at Brown Elementary School, they had a schoolwide Checker Tournament and Chess Tournament and Mark won both of them.

He joined Cub Scouts when he was eight and continued until he made Arrow of Light, the highest award in Cub Scouts. He worked and worked on his badges. Once he started something, he would keep at it.

Whether it was a Little League game or just a game of "Monopoly," he played his hardest. He loved cards and, having a name like Hoyle, he had to. He used to beat every visitor that would play him in "Connect Four." Even some of the nurses would play against him, but Mark always managed to win.

But Mark wasn't up for games on June 11. He was still very weak and being fed intravenously. His blood counts were all very poor. The doctors decided to give him a blood transfusion the next day, which did help his counts a bit.

Thursday, June 13, 1985, we got the worst news of our lives! Mark had AIDS! We thought for sure it was just a bad case of double pneumonia. It never entered our minds that the pneumonia was an effect of AIDS. I guess we really didn't realize how sick our little boy was. My mother would tell me later that she didn't expect him to walk out of that hospital.

Dale cried on my shoulder. We hugged, and I told her that Mark was a fighter. Three times before we had been told Mark might not make it and he always did. We had to have faith in God that everything would work out.

Dale had to leave the hospital. She needed to get some fresh air. I stayed with Mark and tried to answer his questions about our talk with the doctors. Dale and I decided that for the time being, we would not tell Mark about the AIDS diagnosis. It would just depress him, and he needed every bit of strength to fight this pneumonia. It was called pneumocystis carinii, and we had never heard of it before. I told Mark that the doctors now knew what type of pneumonia he had, and that they would start treating him with a drug called Bactrim. He should start feeling better soon. Mark was happy to hear that they definitely knew what he had. "I'm going to get better now, huh Dad?" he asked. I assured him that he would, we made the "thumbs up" sign which was our signal to each other and then gave each other a big hug.

I didn't know where Dale was, and I told Mark that I would find her for him. Meanwhile, I went down to the phone booths on the first floor and called my mother and my mother-in-law. They both were shocked by the bad news but offered to contact other family members for me. I asked them not to tell any of our friends just yet. Later that day I did tell my principal and my boss and friend at Alden Autoparts, where I worked part-time. Sister Martha and Don Grigoreas were both very understanding and caring. The principal told me she would have the whole school pray for Mark. Don told me not to worry about Alden's, the job would be waiting for me when I was ready. I never did go back to it.

Dale also took time off from her part-time job at Sears. She had worked there 10 years—ever since the Swansea Mall opened. She enjoyed her work, but hated being away from the family. One of us was always home with the boys. Dale went to work around 4:15 P.M. a few nights a week and worked about five hours a night. On Saturdays she would have an occasional eight-hour day. I worked Thursday nights and Saturday mornings at Alden's. And every vacation from school, I was there working full-time.

I couldn't find Dale, and so I returned to Mark's intensive care room. My sister Jayne left her work to come see us. She gave me a hug and we just talked, being careful not to let Mark know how sick he really was.

Dale returned and we now noticed something new. All the nurses who attended Mark were now wearing gowns, gloves, and masks over their faces. We were told that the gowns and masks were used to protect Mark. We wondered if this was true, or if they were wearing them to protect themselves from Mark. We were told that all visitors from now on would have to wear the gowns and masks. (Although we did wear the gowns, we never did put on the masks.) Meals were now left outside the room on a little table. All Mark's utensils suddenly became plastic with throwaway plates. Mark wasn't eating anything anyway, but it made us feel like lepers. Signs were put up about "precautions" and all visitors had to go the nurses' desk before being admitted.

It was a monumentally sad day for the Hoyles. My parents, Dale's parents, and many relatives all came to visit, but no one mentioned AIDS. Everyone felt so bad for Mark. My two brothers, Jeff and Jon, just couldn't believe it. Dale's brother and sister, Kenneth and Sue, were also deeply hurt. But we all put on a front and encouraged Mark to get well.

Dr. Mucciardi, Dr. Lemaire, and the residents were all very hopeful. But it was a fairly new illness, and there were still many questions to be answered. The doctors called all over the country getting expert advice from other doctors who had treated AIDS patients. But most of the cases were adult men, not a 12-year-old child. Dr. Mucciardi felt very strongly that Mark could get over this "opportunistic infection" as it was called, but if he came down with it again, it would be much more difficult to fight. I, myself, had no doubts in my mind. I knew he would recover. He had faced death before and always triumphed, he could do it again. He was like a cat with nine lives.

Mark loved cats and at that time we had four: Spooky, Dynamite, Champ, and Dirty. We also had a dog named Cleopatra, Cleo for short, and a 65-gallon aquarium filled with tropical fish. Oh, yes, we had a parakeet named Pretty Boy. Mark certainly did love animals, but cats were his favorite.

The intravenous feedings were keeping Mark from getting any worse, but he still was much too weak to eat. Dale even tried to bribe him to eat by offering him a dollar a bite. This was one offer he could not refuse. He always wanted extra money to buy baseball cards. He had lost a lot of weight and was down to just 70 pounds. It pleased us both to see him eating even a few bites again. We would have bought him anything he asked for, but he just wasn't hungry.

Baseball cards were the perfect gift for Mark. He was an avid collector. He often talked about opening a card shop when he was older. Mark read everything there was to read on the subject of baseball cards and he seemed to know the price of every card ever made. He collected complete sets, special sets, favorite players, and the Red Sox. He loved autographed cards and spent a great deal of time writing away to baseball stars. He also wrote to movie stars, TV personalities, newscasters, and others asking for autographed pictures. Whether quickly or months later, most people responded, and Mark's collection grew steadily.

By 1986 he had stopped writing personal letters. Instead he had me run off copies of a letter for him. It said: "Dear _____, My name is Mark Hoyle. I am 13 years old and collect autographs. It is an interesting hobby. I would love to add your autograph to my collection. Could you please sign these cards for me or if you can't, could you please send me an autographed picture of yourself. Thanks for considering my request. Sincerely, Mark."

Now, even after his death, we are still getting autographed cards made out to Mark. He always enclosed a stamped, self-addressed envelope. It is very strange receiving mail in Mark's handwriting.

Getting back to June of 1985, the Bactrim did start to show signs of working. It took a few days to notice a change, but Mark did seem to be getting stronger. He did start to get his appetite back, but his blood counts were still very low. He was able to come off the oxygen which he had really needed for a few days. But then on the eighth day of the Bactrim, he started to get sick again. He started to get a rash and he was vomiting. The doctors had warned us that this might happen. They originally said that most patients with pneumocystis carinii were on Bactrim for 14 days. They wanted Mark to be on it for 21 days. But here it was only his eighth day and he was allergic to it. The doctors told us that there was another drug that could be used—pentamidine. Hopefully, Mark wouldn't be allergic to this, too.

Father's Day was June 16 that year and my birthday was June 18. Mark was well enough to make me two beautiful cards. I really treasured those cards, but couldn't enjoy either day.

The pentamidine was started, another IV drug. Mark made a calendar going back to June 10, the day he was admitted. The days passed slowly and it was very hot. Mark's room was not air-conditioned, he didn't have much of a view from his bed, and he was starting to get bored with the place. This was a good sign; he was getting well again. The nurses couldn't believe all the cards he was getting. We put them on the door from top to bottom and soon we had to start on the walls, too. Everyone brought him gifts until it seemed that there was no place left to put them. Dale and I were still alternating nights at the hospital, sleeping on a fold-up cot in Mark's room.

One of our friends, the Medeiros family, knew someone who knew Kelly Tripucka, then with the Detroit Pistons. He sent one of his own basketball shirts for Mark. On the front he wrote in marker: "To Mark Hoyle, Keep on Fighting, Always! Kelly Tripucka #7." This really cheered him up and we displayed it on the wall for all visitors to see.

Another happy time was when Russ Gibson came up to see Mark. He and his son Chris brought Mark an autographed ball. Since the Red Sox were his favorite team, meeting the former catcher was a big thrill. The ball was marked: "To Mark, I'm proud of you. Keep fighting. I wish you the best. Your friend, Russ Gibson '67 Sox." He took off his World Series ring from '67 and Mark tried it on for size. It didn't quite fit. Later Mark would ask, "Did you see the size of his hands? Wow, he's a big guy!" Russ also promised to get him a few autographs of the San Francisco Giants. He was going to a reunion in California and would be meeting with some of his old buddies. (Russ had also played for the Giants.) When he got back he came to our house with an autographed ball signed by about 15 members of the '71 Giants. He also had an autographed picture of Willie McCovey.

Another special time for Mark was when his Little League manager and coach, Reggie Desnoyers and Leo Roy, sneaked up to see him. They brought him greetings from the whole team and a ball signed by everyone. It meant a great deal to Mark.

Father Jim Fitzpatrick from St. John Church in Attleboro also came to visit. He brought with him over 300 "schoolmade" greeting cards for Mark from the students at St. John's. He really enjoyed reading them, especially the ones from grade one.

June 24 made it exactly two weeks that Mark was in the hospital. He was feeling much better, but was still a long way from complete recovery. He used to sit near the window and talk to some of the kids from the neighborhood who would walk by.

He never gave them his real name, he told them his name was "George." Different kids would call up to him by this name. His room was on the second floor. Many of my nephews and nieces would also go across the street from the hospital so they could see Mark in the window. He enjoyed talking to them like this.

His brother Scott would also come for a visit depending on which head nurse was on duty. Scott wasn't supposed to visit because of his age. They couldn't talk by phone, because Mark didn't have one in his room. But they did give each other messages on tape. Here is an example transcribed from the tapes:

(Scott talking after he sang a little introduction) "To Mark Hoyle in the hospital. I hope you get my dollar that I gave you when I sent you the card. I know you're sick and I was feeling terrible the other day, too. My head was hot, and my foot was paining me and everything. At home Champ misses you and so do all the other cats. Not much is new here. But our grass looks awful and high. And the cats are praying for you all day long while they sleep and rest. Mom hasn't changed a bit. She's still cleaning all around here. Your cat misses you so much and says he wants to jump all over you when you get home. Mark, I know you're bored, and I'm making this tape especially for you. It was all my idea. I don't have that much more to say to you, so I better say good-bye. I hope you enjoyed this tape. It took me a long time to prepare this. I'll see you, good luck, hope you feel better, bye. But don't forget your cat, little Champypoo, is praying for you, so don't give up! Your little kitty will be so happy when you show up at home."

(Mark talking) "Hello, Scott. How are you doing? Right now I'm pretty bored up here. I'm just lying in bed in the hospital. Pretty soon it's going to be midnight. Right now it's 11:55 P.M. Well, there's nothing much to say. I liked your tape about Champ. Believe me, Scott, you wouldn't want to be up here. It's a big pain! I had to have a new medicine put into me today, and now my right arm, where I get treatment, had 16 shots and it's all swollen. And every 15 minutes at night they have to wake me up to take my blood pressure, put the stethoscope on my heart, and they almost put the ET finger on me. That makes my whole finger turn red. But I'm starting to feel better.

"I wiped Dad out at checkers and I wiped Papa out, too. The score with Dad is nine to three and I'm ahead. Tonight I wiped him out wicked bad. I played him three games and won all three. We quit because Papa and Nana came. Papa wanted to play me and I beat him twice and then he quit. Then I had my ice cream sundae. I'm starting to eat a little more, but I still have to have all these medicines, and I can't move around too much.

"I'm getting a lot of cards. All my flowers are dying. I don't have a good TV with cable like you have. I wish I was home— you're so lucky! Going around to Nana's house and doing all kinds of good stuff. I wish I was lucky like that. But one of my lungs is completely healed and the other one is better. But there's nothing to really do here. I've been playing this airplane game called 'Emperor.' What have you been doing lately? Nothing much? What about at home? Does Dad give the cats a lot of milk? I hope he does. You should just enjoy life as you can. I hope your toe feels better, too. Dad said you stepped on something and your whole foot was sore. You had to lay down all the time. I really feel bad for you. I hope you get better soon. I heard you got double treatment one day. I think you stayed at Nana Hoyle's for a while. Have you seen any good movies lately? 20, 19, 18, 17, 16, 15, 14, 13, 12, 11, 10, 9, 8, 7, 6, 5, 4, 3, 2, 1 YEAH! It's midnight! It's exactly midnight right now.

"I planned this tape for a long time. I hope you like it. I just wanted to say that we're so lucky to have Mom and Dad. They're so nice to us, huh? I hope you're not mad at me because you think I'm getting all the attention. But, I'm not, I'm not, Scott. You're so lucky too, because you get to see the two Nanas all the time, and travel. I wish I could just be outside for 10 minutes, just 10 minutes! I did get to go for a ride down to X-ray today. It's pretty scary seeing all the machines and everything. When I got back, I fell and almost killed myself trying to get from the cot to my bed. Well, that's how things are.

"Today I was watching TV most of the day and I took a nap. Last night, I woke up with a nosebleed—at midnight. Me and Dad stayed awake until 2 o'clock, because I just couldn't sleep. I was trying to. Finally, at 2 o'clock, I told Dad to go to bed, so he did. But I was still awake and kept looking at the clock. Finally at 2:30, he looked at me and said, 'What are you still doing awake?' And I told him I wasn't tired. So, at 3 o'clock, I was still awake and woke Dad up because I had to go to the bathroom. Finally I got to sleep around quarter of 4. And then at 4, they came in and woke me up to take my blood pressure again. What a pain! And I couldn't get to sleep until 4:15. It was a terrible night, but I slept late this morning. They let me sleep until 10:30. I watched 'Sale of the Century' and then the 'Price is Right.' Later I had a cruddy Dunkin Donut. I like Bess Eaton better. Then I had a salad for lunch and went to sleep. Then Nana and Tony came. Later I went down to X-ray.

"Well, I hope your foot feels better. I've got to be going because it's too late now. OK? I love you Scotty. Even though you're my brother, could you do me a favor? Could you please take care of my cat? Bye Scott. Byeeeeeeee. Bye Scott. See you later Scott. Bye. Bye. Bye. Bye. Byeeeeeeeeee."

(*Scott talking*) "To my wonderful brother Mark, from his 'bro' Scott. I liked your tape about everything. It's true about Dunkin Donuts, even though I didn't try their jimmies yet. The grass once again looks very atrocious and Stephen forgot to mow it. I heard about my foot on your tape. My foot is better, but I don't think I'll make practice Sunday because I don't think it's that much better yet because it's only a little bit swollen. My left foot is better, but my right foot is still a little bit swollen. Dad taped *The Natural* for you. It took him a long time to do it. It was on at 10 o'clock and was over at 12:18 — that's two hours and 18 minutes that movie is. So, you'll have to watch it because Dad stayed up a long time and Dad was very tired.

"Well, I'll get back to you in a minute because I have to give your kitty some milk. Everybody is taking care of your favorite kitty. He's staying in every night and I'm giving him lots of milk. He misses you though, but when you get back, he's going to go with you — sleep with you all night and still I'm giving him milk #1, I'm giving him food #2, and #3 I'm petting him all the time. He sleeps in my bed, sleeps in Dad's bed, sleeps on your bed, he sleeps on everything — even the couch. I always pet him, cuddle him at night, and make sure he's inside for you, especially for you, and my cat is doing good also. My cat is softer than ever, cuter than ever, fluffier than ever and fatter

than ever. It still sucks on things though. That's the bad news
about my cat Tiger. The good part is that he likes me. Your cat
is always playing with my cat and they wrestle a lot. The kitties are so funny when you look at them—when they fight
wrestle. Before I go to bed I always look for your cat—to make
sure that he's in. If he's not in, I'll go to both doors and I'll call
him for 15 minutes. And by that time he should be coming.
I'll always do this especially for you, Mark, because you're sick.
And because you asked me to, but I'm doing it anyway because
I like you—a lot! . . .

"I am trying to think of things to say because not much is
happening around here, except that I miss you and so does
Mom, Dad, Champ, Tiger, Dirty, and Spooky, and don't forget
my parakeet, the fish, and don't forget Cleo! Cleo is getting
older and older. All she does is sit around all day and sleep.
Sometimes she sleeps with her eyes open. I wish I could bring
Champ to you. You would be so happy to see him. I know how
much you miss him. And I hope you like my tape—the one
with the kitties and everything—and the pictures. Mom was
only going to take one picture, but I said, 'Mom, take two pictures.' And I did that just for you so you can have two pictures
of Champ to look at. I hope you liked it all. Well, I'm going to
eat now. Byeeeee.

"Now I'm back. I already ate. Now I'm full after that chicken
noodle soup I had. You think I have it easy. You thought wrong!
It's not easy going to everyone's house and having to walk around
on sore feet. Going to the bathroom is especially hard.

"Yesterday I played with Shane. Yesterday was Friday and we
played 'Atari.' I creamed him in baseball. Tell me what you've
been eating in the hospital on your next tape. I'll tell you what
I've been having. (Scott spent about five minutes going through
his weekly meals.)

"And I hope you give me another tape. It will be like pen pals.
Try to make the tape soon.

"I hope you feel better with your double pneumonia and
everything. I heard that one lung is completely better and one
isn't as good, but almost better. But I hope that other lung is
better soon so you can have fun like old times, like play baseball in the yard or something. That would be fun! But my foot
is not completely healed and neither are you. Oh well! I miss

you, Mark. I love you and hope you feel better. I'll be seeing you, good luck, byeeee."

(*Mark talking*) "How are you? How are you? How are you? (then Mark sang "10 Little Indians") Hi Scott the Wot. Having fun? I'm not having fun right now. They woke me up early to get on the scale. I was wicked, wicked tired. By the way, I got a shirt. Guess who the guy is who gave it to me! Kelly Tripucka! (*siren*) Hear that noise? That's the cops. They just went flying by. There's really not that much to do right now. Mom's up with me right now. I did get a lot of money. If I win the Megabucks tonight, I'll give you some. If I win $40, I'll give you $5, Dad $5, and Mom $5. Is that fair? That's a lot of money, huh? And thanks for the dollar you gave me, it made me very happy knowing it was your own money.

"When I get out I'm going to pet the cats so much. I can't wait to put my hands all along Champ's back. The doctors said I might get out around July 3. (He didn't.) That's in eight more days—that's a long time, but it's better than two weeks from now. Hey Scott, guess what? Mom said that when I get out, we're going to go everywhere. Wherever I want to go we can go. And by the way, you know the den, that's going to be your room. Soon as I get out of here we're going to start making some changes. So why don't you start making plans? Draw the room on a piece of paper and put things where they're going to go like your bed, bureau, and everything else. You know what I mean jellybean? Ha Ha Ha!

"How you doing, Scotty? Wherever you are, where are you— home? At one of the Nanas' houses? Where are you? Tell me, tell me, please! How's Cleo doing? Have you seen Spooky lately? By the way, I got a fruit basket. There's all kinds of fruit like bananas, apples, green apples, pineapples, nectarines. What else is there, Mom? Grapes, peaches, plums—hey man, we've been talking a long time. It's about time we shortened it up. Remember, I want to see your plans for your new room. I already made one for my bedroom. OK? So make your plans. It's almost time for lunch, I have yucky stuff! It tastes like garbage! It probably tastes like garbage because it is. Ha Ha! Hey Scott, I'm getting a lot of cards. The whole door is full now. I have my shirt hanging on the other door. Isn't that a funny place for it? I got out of bed and did a little dance for Mom. I couldn't get back into the bed because I had it raised so high. It must have been four and one-half feet high. That's a long way up. Well, I have to go because my lunch is here."

July 1 came and went and we started making plans for the 4th of July. We got permission to bring Mark to the game room so we could watch the fireworks that were held at the nearby Kennedy Park. They made Mark wear a mask when he moved from his room to the game room—a distance of no more than 20 feet. We had this whole room to ourselves. Mark was thrilled to get out of his room. Dale, Mark, and I sat by the window and really enjoyed the display. Scott went with my parents to watch them in person. Later, we had permission from Nancy Harkness to light some sparklers out the window. Nancy is a social worker who was very helpful to our whole family during this trying period at St. Anne's. She has since become a very close friend. The only trouble with the sparklers was the breeze brought the smoke into the room and we thought it was going to set the fire alarm off. Mark loved it—he laughed and laughed.

All the doctors from Pediatrics were so nice. They would come and visit Mark every day. Dr. Rock even won a ticket for a balloon ride which he gave to Mark. Then Mark gave it to me for my birthday. When the big day came, it was too windy. I was really glad! Dr. Sheehan, another pulmonary expert, also visited Mark quite a bit. Everyone who met Mark liked him. He always seemed to bring out the best in people. When he became healthier, he started playing practical jokes on the nurses. Mark loved a good joke.

Mark started to get ill again and so the doctors took him off the pentamidine. He soon was better and getting more and more restless. On Friday, July 5, we were able to walk down the hall and go out on a patio. Mark loved the fresh air. It was a great change for him.

His blood counts were still low, but the X-rays showed his lungs were clear. He felt great! On Saturday, July 6, around 7 P.M., Dr. Penn came in and asked Mark if he wanted to go home. Mark said, "Yes," and he said, "OK." It was a big surprise because earlier we had been told that Mark's blood counts would have to go up before he could go home. Mark had spent 27 days and 26 nights at the hospital.

All the way home he appreciated all the little things that we take for granted. The trees, the sky, the clouds all meant so much to him. He was really excited to be home. He hugged his animals and we brought in all the items that he had accumulated while in the hospital. "I love you, Mom and Dad," he said. "Thanks for staying with me all that time."

Mark was home. But now came the hard part. How would I tell my son that he had AIDS? We decided it could wait a while longer until Mark was more healthy.

It was great to have Mark home. He was looking forward to sleeping in his own bed again. Scott and Mark both shared a bedroom and one of the things we promised Mark was that when he got better, he could have his own room. Mark looked forward to this and had drawn up many plans while in the hospital. The move would have to be made right away. But before we could do this, we had to reorganize several rooms and closets and furnishings.

Soon it was time for the big move. Furniture, toys, books, baseball cards, etc., were everywhere. The house was a mess! Then the phone rang. It was Nancy Harkness, the social worker from St. Anne's. She wanted to come over for a visit. We welcomed her to our messy, upside down house. We were embarrassed, but promised her that on her next visit everything would be in order again.

Mark and Scott each took control of their own rooms. They designed them in their own tastes and everything came out fine. Mark decided to put his autographed pictures on the walls over his bed. He bought plastic pages for all his autographed cards and pictures and they filled two walls. The rest of his cards were neatly arranged in looseleaf folders by year. He labeled everything and kept his extra cards in his drawers.

Mark was the type who would send away for 50 of one particular card because he'd say "that card is going to be worth money some day." He loved his hobby and spent a great deal of time on it.

Meanwhile, Dale and I were reading everything we could get our hands on about AIDS. The articles said there were no specific symptoms for AIDS. But some symptoms that appear are probably due to low-grade infections that occur because a person's immune system is defective. We tried to think back about any symptoms Mark might have shown. He did show extreme fatigue, he did have headaches, and he did have a persistent fever throughout May and June. He hadn't shown any signs of shaking chills and night sweats at that particular time. (Later on he did have these symptoms along with terrible nightmares that certain creatures were trying to get him.)

One symptom is a 10–20 pound weight loss within a few months and Mark did seem to lose about 10 pounds. Swollen lymph glands were another of his symptoms, but he had had these many times before. General aches and pains and a feeling of illness for more than 10 days is another of the symptoms that Mark certainly had.

Dale and I were aware of all these symptoms before Mark became sick because we belonged to both the Rhode Island Hemophilia Foundation and the New England Hemophilia Association. Both organizations sent out frequent updates about AIDS. But the symptoms listed seemed like symptoms for any virus and I just never even thought of Mark having AIDS. Dale told me later that she feared he had it but didn't say anything. I guess it was her intuition. She feared it, but didn't want to believe it.

We're not sure exactly how he got it. It could have been from a blood transfusion that he had received, or from his factor VIII. More than likely, it was from his factor VIII since he was on every-other-day doses for so long. At any rate, he had it, and now all we could do was pray and hope for a cure.

Mark loved making tents in our backyard. He would put rope between trees and then throw blankets, sheets, afghans, anything he could find to make his lavish shelters. The finished project would look like an Arab's home in the desert with many individual rooms.

It was one of these sunny July days, when Mark was busy making a tent, that I chose to tell him the bad news.

"Mark," I said, "the doctors know what caused you to have that bad case of double pneumonia."

"What?" he asked.

"Mark, it was AIDS."

Tears came to his eyes and he questioned, "Am I going to die, Dad?"

I answered, "Everyone is going to die, Mark; we all have to face death sometime. But you're not going to die now. Look how healthy you are. You don't die just from having AIDS. You die from the infections that you can get from AIDS. And most of these infections are treatable. I have a paper in the house that shows all the treatments they have for the different diseases that people with AIDS can get—they're treatable!"

Trying as best I could to reassure him, I continued, "I know, Mark, that this is terrible and scary news. But I also know you're a fighter. I know you can beat this thing. If God wanted you to die, He could have taken you at St. Anne's Hospital. Look how sick you were. Look how healthy you feel now.

"I just have a feeling that everything's going to be all right. They're working on a cure now, I'm sure they'll find one soon." Mark gave me his usual tight hug.

He was very quiet. He went back to working on his tent. Dale came out and I told her that Mark knew. She also encouraged him. We both promised him that we would back him 100%. Any time he had to go in the hospital, one of us would always be there. But for now, we would just worry about him getting stronger and healthier.

I felt drained. Dr. Smith had wanted Mark to know and finally I had done it. It wasn't easy. But I think it was the right thing to do. What if he had found out from someone else? He never would have trusted us again. It was the thing to do, and I did it.

The summer passed quickly. Mark became stronger and stronger each day. His appetite was back to normal and he was gaining some weight back. We had weekly blood tests at St. Anne's Hospital and then usually had breakfast together in the park.

Mark was well enough to take golf lessons at Montaup Country Club in Portsmouth, Rhode Island. My father was club secretary and he arranged for Mark, Scott, and the rest of his grandchildren to take the weekly lessons. There were about 50 children taking these lessons.

Both our boys did very well. Scott even won a contest when he got a hole-in-one while chipping from 10 feet off the green. At the last lesson, the pro used his videocamera to take pictures of all the children. We had a copy made and it's a joy to watch.

Later, Mark was able to go back to Little League for the final two games. He didn't get any hits, but he played flawlessly in the field. His teammates were all glad to have him back. I think he felt bad that he didn't hit well but at least he was back on the diamond playing the game he loved so much.

Mark was able to mow the lawn, rake, and work in the yard. He loved working with wood and he helped me make a couple of decks in the backyard. He would go with me to Grossman's and help pick out the wood. He was a big help to me.

He also got the idea for a tree house. We worked on it together. It's about 12 feet off the ground and has a door, but no roof. It was supposed to be for both Mark and Scott, but we ended up putting up another tree house in another tree for Scott.

Besides these backyard projects, Mark also played baseball with the neighborhood kids and rode his bicycle. He also loved shooting baskets and playing street hockey. Of course we went to flea markets every week so the kids could buy baseball cards and Dale could search for bargains.

We went duckpin bowling, miniature golfing, and had a pretty busy summer. It was a very healthy summer for Mark. Even though for the first time ever we did not go on a family vacation, we spent as much time together as we could—especially in our above-ground pool.

We also made trips to Providence to see Dr. Smith. It was weekly at first, then every two weeks, and then every month.

It was at one of these appointments that we discussed school. Dr. Mucciardi had said that there was no reason for Mark not to go. We asked Dr. Smith what he thought. He agreed with Dr. Mucciardi. It would be best for Mark to continue to do all his normal activities. Dale and I were worried about Mark picking something up in school. But Dr. Smith told us that there were germs everywhere and Mark would have just as much of a chance of picking them up at home. His idea was to keep Mark healthy—exercising, eating properly, getting the proper amount of rest, etc.

We had read a great deal about AIDS and knew Mark couldn't give it to anyone by casual contact. The doctors all told us the same thing. That's why we had no fear of Mark giving AIDS to someone in school. At home we never broke the regular routine. We continued to act the way we always acted. We hugged Mark, kissed him, drank out of the same glass with him, shared utensils, etc. Dale and I continued to mix his factor VIII treatment without using gloves and we helped give his treatment. His grandmothers and aunts continued to kiss and hug him and no one treated him any differently. We tried to make life as normal as possible for Mark. He played with his brother and the neighborhood kids. Friends came over to our house and on his 13th birthday, August 2, we took a group of his friends miniature golfing and then had cake and ice cream.

The one thing that was different about Mark was his questions about God. He had more and more of them as time passed. He was always religious, even working for and receiving a religious award in Cub Scouts, but AIDS seemed to bring out his love of God even more. At night especially he would pray for the longest time before going to bed. Once I asked him what he said to God. He explained how he prayed for his family, relatives, friends, and everyone in the world. He prayed that his brother would not get AIDS. He told me that he started praying to God about this when the news of AIDS first came out in the newspapers.

He had many questions about heaven, and often asked me what I thought it would be like. The topic intrigued him, but he wasn't obsessed with it. Mark learned a great deal about religion from Dale and me. Dale belonged to the First Christian Congregationalist Church and I belonged to St. Dominic's Catholic Church. Many Sundays we would go to her service at 10 o'clock and then go to my mass at 11:30.

I found myself also wondering about God. And I started to ask Him many questions. But deep down inside I really believed that God would cure Mark and everything was going to be all right. I started praying to St. Jude, saint of the impossible. I made novenas and put holy water on Mark. We had some friends give us water from Lourdes, LaSalette, Our Lady of Knock in Ireland, and St. Anne's in Canada. I prayed to St. James, my patron saint, I prayed to St. Francis (my middle name is Francis), I prayed to St. Mark, I prayed to the Infant of Prague, and I prayed to Mary. I prayed to the relatives of mine who had died, I prayed to Dale's relatives who had died. I prayed for a cure. "Ask and you shall receive" I had been taught. God wouldn't let me down. Not a teacher from a Catholic school who really believed in His mission. Not a person who always wore the scapular of Mary and still does. I had the family pray together and put our hands on Mark. We prayed, Mark seemed healthier, and I was happy.

We went to my school in August to decorate the room. It had been a family tradition that we all went to Attleboro and pitched in to get the job done. The boys seemed to enjoy doing this. Mark brought his friend Bobby Evans.

As we drove back to Swansea, we passed LaSalette Shrine. Everyone noticed the sign stretching across the roadway. It advertised the upcoming fair for Labor Day weekend. Mark and Scott always enjoyed going each year. They would try their skill at the many games and their luck on others. We promised we would go up again.

Mark was actually pretty healthy that August. We took his temperature daily and the average came out to be 99.7. We always took his temperature shortly after he woke up and usually another two or three times during the day. He hated this, but we wanted to be aware of any infection that he might catch so that it could be treated immediately. His blood counts were still low and would continue to stay low during his entire illness. His white blood count was 1700 on August 20, 1985, while his hemoglobin was a low 8.9. I always liked statistics and kept accurate records of his temperatures and blood counts throughout his illness, as well as the number of bleeds and factor VIII used.

Even though Mark didn't have any problems relating to AIDS the rest of the summer of 1985, he still had problems with his hemophilia. He needed eight vials of factor VIII in July. These were for nosebleeds, a right shoulder injury, a hematoma on his left thigh, and right ankle problems.

August was worse. He needed 12 vials of factor VIII, mostly

for a right ankle problem. His ankles and right elbow had always been problem joints. Many times when Mark was younger he would cry out in pain from the swelling in those three joints. But his ankles had been fine since July 31. All of August he walked perfectly with no problems until the 26th. It was that day, my mother's birthday, the day before school started, that his ankle started acting up.

Scott also had bleeding problems during Mark's illness. I had to give him 12 treatments in May due to problems with his left knee and right ankle. In June, Scott had 16 treatments for his right ankle, right elbow, and right foot. July was worse, Scott received 32 treatments—all for his left knee. He was put in a cast at Lakeville Hospital and had a miserable month. August came and Scott had 15 treatments—again, all for the left knee. Wasn't life fun?

2

"I think they should just leave him alone and let him go to school."

—Eighth grader Ronnie Parker

D
r. Smith was on vacation and didn't realize that Swansea started school earlier than most schools. They always started a week before Labor Day. The original purpose for the early opening was to permit schools to be closed during the winter for a longer period of time and thereby save on heating expenses. Since Labor Day in 1985 was September 2, Swansea's schools would open Tuesday, August 27. Dr. Smith did not find this out until our visit with him on August 20.

Dr. Smith called John E. McCarthy, superintendent of schools, and Harold Devine, principal of Case Junior High School, to set up a meeting for Monday morning, August 26. This was the day before school was to begin. Nothing was mentioned over the phone about Mark's illness.

Mr. McCarthy had heard rumors about Mark and called us about a week before this meeting. Dale confirmed the rumors that, yes, Mark had AIDS. We had nothing to hide. It wasn't a big secret. By now we had told all our relatives and friends, the Little League coaches, and anyone else who we thought ought to know. I never asked where he heard the rumors, but some people had told me that people from St. Anne's Hospital who lived in Swansea had been talking. It didn't really matter to us who told. My wife talked to the superintendent about 20 minutes. He explained that he would be looking into the subject more and would get back to us. Dale seemed very pleased talking to him. She thought he seemed very nice and very fair.

Mr. McCarthy would later say, "I knew nothing about AIDS. I didn't know what to do nor what we had to do. I was like the average person in Swansea who had very little knowledge about

26

the fatal disease." He immediately began researching the topic. He turned to the experts at the state departments of Education and Public Health. He called the Federal Centers for Disease Control (CDC) in Atlanta, Georgia. They told him that "for most infected school-age children, the benefits of an unrestricted setting (i.e., school) would outweigh the apparent nonexistent risk of transmission of the AIDS virus." All the official agencies gave Superintendent McCarthy the same findings—"a child has the right to attend public school, unless a physician determines otherwise." Dr. George Grady, the Massachusetts epidemiologist, also had the same response.

I asked Dr. Smith if I should plan on attending the meeting with the superintendent that was scheduled for Monday, August 26. He said that Dale and I were certainly welcome. But Dale was nervous about going and chose not to attend. I knew that Dr. Smith would be accompanied by Nancy Keyes, R.N., and Debra DeMaio, M.S.W. Nancy was the head nurse in the hemophilia program at Rhode Island Hospital and Debbie was the hemophilia social worker. Both were also good friends. What I didn't expect was the number of people from the school faculty. In addition to Superintendent McCarthy and Mr. Devine, all the teachers who would have Mark that year were at the meeting. There must have been at least 14 people counting gym, music, art, cooking, health, woodshop, metal shop, and all the major subjects. The lawyer for the school department was also present as were the school physician and nurse.

Dr. Smith gave an excellent presentation on why Mark belonged in school. He said that Mark would not be endangering anyone in the school and it was the proper place for him to be. Nancy Keyes and Debbie DeMaio also made short presentations and then all three answered questions from the audience. I was also called upon to answer a question about Mark's health that summer. I told them how he had completely recovered from the pneumonia, was feeling great, and had even gone back and played Little League baseball. He had taken golf lessons also, and no one had treated him differently, including his friends.

The school physician seemed to have the most questions and the meeting went on for quite some time. At the end of the meeting Superintendent McCarthy told the group that he would have his decision about Mark's attendance by the end of the day.

After the meeting I thanked Dr. Smith, Nancy Keyes, and Debbie DeMaio and went home to tell Dale about the large turnout. She was surprised also. We had thought that maybe Swansea would follow the lead of Kokomo, Indiana. It was there that Ryan White, a hemophiliac who had contracted AIDS, was not allowed to attend school. His story had made headlines across the U.S. We really hoped that we could keep Mark's health problem a secret from the press. It was hard enough dealing with AIDS without dealing with the public, too. We wanted to protect Mark and let him lead as full a life as possible. Mark was always a quiet boy and we didn't know how all this would affect him.

The day seemed to drag as we waited for Mr. McCarthy's phone call. Mark's ankle became worse and worse. He had such bad luck. He always seemed to get a bleed at the worst possible time. It looked like he would have to start the school year on crutches. Yes, the call came and we were thrilled to learn that Mark would be allowed in school. We wanted Mark to be what he was—a 13-year-old boy who was going to school. Mark seemed happy, too, although he had said if they wouldn't let him go, he'd enjoy staying in bed in the morning and watching TV all day.

Tuesday, August 27, Mark went to school on crutches. It's hard on any child that age to have to go like that. You feel like everyone is looking at you. But Mark went and, except for the fact that his ankle hurt him, he had a good day. We picked him up at noon because we didn't want to let him get too tired.

We had given him his needle in the morning and decided to give him another dose at night. His right ankle was becoming more swollen and painful.

Wednesday, August 28, Mark received two doses of factor VIII before school. We only had him go until noon again and picked him up at the office. By nighttime, his ankle seemed a little better.

Thursday, August 29, Dr. Smith held an after-school meeting with the full faculty, Mr. McCarthy, and Mr. Devine. Rumors had spread about the boy with AIDS and so it was necessary to discuss the issue. The meeting lasted for three hours. Debbie DeMaio told us that it was a very emotional meeting. There were many questions and sincere concerns expressed. But by the end of the meeting, it seemed to her that the staff had accepted Dr. Smith's reassurances. Mr. Devine was quoted as saying, "It was the faculty members who had attended the first meeting who should be credited with making the outcome so positive. Those teachers were secure in their understanding of the situation and helped the others to understand. They had an opportunity to resolve their personal crises, were in support of what was happening. They more or less teamed up with Dr. Smith in order to reassure their colleagues." There were a few teachers who were still opposed to Mark's attendance. One teacher was so fearful he transferred to the high school.

WLNE, a Providence, Rhode Island, television station, and the *Providence Journal-Bulletin* contacted the school department about rumors that an AIDS victim was attending school in Swansea. Mr. Devine was also contacted but would not confirm the story. He told me that he would not cooperate with them. He reminded them of all the protests going on in Indiana, New York, and elsewhere by parents opposed to schoolchildren with AIDS. The reporters were also told that they would bear a "heavy responsibility" if they ran stories that were unconfirmed. The two news organizations listened to Mr. Devine and did not run the story.

On Thursday and Friday Mark again went until noon. I picked him up at the office because I hadn't started school yet. I had taken the summer off for the first time since I was in high school. Mark was only using one crutch so it was easier for him to carry his books. He had treatment both days.

Saturday Mark's ankle was much better. We promised him we would go to the LaSalette Fair the next day. He received one treatment and was in a great mood. He had gone to school for four days with AIDS, and no one even mentioned it to him. He was just one of the students in the eighth grade. And that's the way he wanted it.

LaSalette was fun for both of the boys. They loved playing the games of chance and the money spent went to a good cause. John Ghiorse, the TV weatherman, was in one of the booths and Mark enjoyed seeing him in person. There were plenty of rides and food. Mark won a "Playboy" mirror which is now hanging above our bar in the family room. I said that it was funny that you go to a religious fair and end up winning a "Playboy" item. They also won many trinkets and some goldfish. I ran into some old students from St. John's and some present students. We also bumped into many other people we knew. Mark was able to walk pretty well. We did not give him treatment.

Monday, September 2, was Labor Day. We gave him a prophylactic treatment just to make sure the ankle didn't swell up again. Mark said it felt fine but he agreed he should get one as a precaution. We also gave one to him on Tuesday, before school.

As the day went on that Tuesday, Mark's ankle started to bother him again. By Wednesday, September 4, he needed two vials of treatment. Wednesday was also a day that we'll never forget. The local weekly newspaper, *The Spectator*, published a front page article with the heading: "No decision yet on school attendance for stricken child." It also mentioned that "Swansea records one case of AIDS." The article, written by Barbara Davies, had up-to-date information about AIDS but didn't say anything else about Mark. However, the headline was inaccurate since Mark had been attending school with permission.

On Thursday morning the *Providence Journal* came out with a front page article under the headline: "Swansea student, AIDS victim, attends school with official OK." It was written by Irene Wielawski with reports from W. Zachary Malinowski and Bob Jagolinzer. The story went on to say how a "teenage boy, suffering from AIDS as a result of treatment for hemophilia has, with the permission of school officials, quietly been attending Case Junior High School since school began Aug. 27." The article continued:

> The decision to admit him was based on his doctor's assurances that normal school contact would not lead to transmission of the deadly and incurable acquired immune deficiency syndrome. The case appears to be the first in the nation in which a child with AIDS has knowingly been allowed into a public school system.
>
> The situation came to light after teachers anonymously contacted the *Journal-Bulletin* to express continuing ap-

prehension about the possibility of catching AIDS through casual contact with the boy.

Swansea School Supt. John E. McCarthy and the boy's doctor, Dr. Peter Smith of Rhode Island Hospital in Providence, confirmed yesterday that he is attending school.

McCarthy said Swansea school officials decided not to inform parents of other children at the junior high in order to protect the boy's privacy.

"Confidentiality," McCarthy said, "that's not only my view, that's the law. God help us for that kid."

School Committee Chairman Robert Paquette declined to comment. Committeeman James Carvalho said, "The School Committee has been advised by legal counsel not to comment on it."

The case contrasts with a similar and widely publicized situation in Kokomo, Ind., in which a 13-year-old hemophiliac AIDS victim, Ryan White, was barred from school last month by order of the local school superintendent.

Teachers and most parents in the Indiana case sided with the superintendent, and a federal court refused to hear the White family's appeal. The boy has been forced to monitor his classes from home by means of a video camera and telephone hookup. By contrast, four Swansea teachers interviewed yesterday were uniformly supportive of the boy, and said they had been convinced by Dr. Smith that AIDS could not be spread through normal contact among schoolchildren.

Evidence so far indicates that the virus associated with AIDS, known as HTLV-III, is spread through intimate sexual contact and the mingling of body fluids such as blood or semen.

Hemophiliacs are at risk for the disease because they depend on clotting agents derived from thousands of pints of donated blood.

Until the virus was identified a year ago, blood banks were unable to screen donations for HTLV-III contamination so hemophiliacs unknowingly became infected through the clotting concentrates used to control their potentially fatal bleeding disorder.

The Federal Centers for Disease Control recommended recently that children with AIDS be permitted to attend school if they do not have open sores or behavior traits that increase the chances of transmission—such as biting or inability to control their bowels.

Massachusetts health and education officials disclosed yesterday that they are formulating similar guidelines for the state's public schools. The proposal is currently under review by the governor's task force on AIDS and by Education Commissioner John Lawson.

Dr. Smith declined to answer any questions specifically relating to the boy's condition, citing the confidentiality of medical records. But he agreed to be interviewed yesterday about his efforts to defuse any hostility the boy might encounter as a result of what Smith perceives as widespread fear and misunderstanding of AIDS.

Smith said he met with Swansea school officials in midsummer to address any questions or fears they might have concerning the boy's medical condition.

The meeting involved the principal of the school, Harold Devine, the school nurse and a "small number of teachers who would be directly involved in the instruction of this child," Smith said. Also present were the boy's father and a social worker and nurse from the hemophilia center.

At the request of school administrators, Smith said, he met again last week with a larger group of teachers and staff at Case Junior High who wanted to raise questions they apparently were reluctant to ask in the presence of the boy's father.

"There must have been 30 or 40 people there," Smith said. "The nature of it was to go over concerns the teachers had, and to go over questions. It went on for a very long time."

Smith said he perceived "lots of fear" in the group.

"I had the feeling that there was a certain amount of not wanting to accept the unlikeliness of AIDS being passed on," he said. "A few got up and said, 'There is no way you can assure me that there is no possible way I can get this.'

"I answered that there is no way you can give that assurance," Smith recounted. "In the biological sciences, there is no such thing as 100 percent. But I also said: 'You face greater risk getting into an automobile. And I can't promise you that no one is going to plant a bomb in this school or you are not going to fall out a window.'"

Smith said he did not feel at the end of the meeting that he was successful in calming everyone's fears.

But since then, he said, he has received reports from school administrators and others of a generally supportive attitude toward the boy.

Smith's concerns go beyond the Swansea boy.

As director of the Hemophilia Center of Rhode Island, based at Rhode Island Hospital, Smith supervises the treatment of approximately 80 children and adults, victims of hemophilia in the region.

Because of their dependence on the clotting concentrates, most of his patients are likely to have been exposed to the virus. In spot surveys nationally, 95 percent of severe hemophiliacs have been found to have the HTLV-III antibody in their blood. As many as 20 percent of people who test positive for antibodies are expected to develop AIDS.

The Swansea boy is the first patient at the hemophilia center to develop AIDS, but it is unlikely he will be the last. Smith fears that the boy will become a double victim, ostracized like Ryan White in Indiana.

"I am terribly worried about repercussions," Smith said.

What a way to wake up! You look at the morning paper and find a front page article about your son. Thank God they didn't mention his name! I knew all this publicity would not be good for our family and we agreed not to talk to the press. Dale stayed home with Mark—he couldn't go because he was in a great deal of pain with his ankle again. I gave him two vials of factor VIII before heading to school. Scott went to school as usual.

The afternoon *Fall River Herald-News* also had a front page story about Mark written by Curt Brown and Marcia Pobzeznik. The headline was: "Swansea student has AIDS." It was similar to the *Providence Journal* article, but it had more quotes by public officials in the Department of Education.

The *Herald* also carried Mr. McCarthy's statement under

the heading: "AIDS student permitted to stay in Swansea junior high." Mr. McCarthy's statement was:

> The Swansea School Department reports that a student in the Case Junior High School has been diagnosed as having AIDS. After consultation with medical experts, the Swansea School System elected to continue the child's educational program in the school setting.
>
> The action is consistent with the Department of Education Director, the guidelines published by the Centers for Disease Control (CDC) in Atlanta and the recommendations of the Massachusetts Department of Public Health and the child's attending physician.
>
> The School Department is assured that the continuing attendance of the child at school poses no health risk to any other person.
>
> All the guidelines, as published by the CDC of the United States Department of Health and Human Services, the Public Health Services and the recommendations of the Massachusetts Department of Public Health and the Department of Education, will be followed in dealing with the day to day educational needs of the youngster.
>
> The situation was discussed in detail with the child's physician; Dr. George Grady, the Massachusetts Assistant Commissioner of Health for Laboratories and Communicable Disease Control; Dr. Martha Rogers of the CDC in Atlanta; Curtis Hall, Southeastern Regional Director for the Department of Education.
>
> In recognition of the rights of the student involved, the school department will issue no statement as to the student's identity or provide any other information that would violate the student's rights to confidentiality.

None of the newspapers published Mark's name, setting a precedent that remained unbroken until he died. The TV stations did not give his name either. However, the town was besieged with news reporters that Thursday, September 5. They had helicopters flying over the school and reporters and cameramen running all over the place. Mark's classmates were interviewed while getting onto their buses. Cameras and microphones were being put in parents' faces as they picked up their children. We were amazed when we watched the news that night. We were surprised that none of the students gave out Mark's name.

When I came home that afternoon I found out that TV stations and reporters had been calling Dale for interviews all day. She wouldn't give any and finally took the phone off the hook. Radio talk shows like WALE and WSAR were also discussing our son. Reporters, who were not supposed to know Mark's name, were coming to the house for interviews! The national news stations had also called. What a zoo! My sister Jayne and my brother Jeff came over to offer support.

Boston newspapers also carried the story. The *Globe* had an article similar to the *Providence Journal* story. It also made the front page.

The *Journal* had another front page story on Friday, September 6. The headline was: "Swansea school chief says boy with AIDS will stay." The story by W. Zachary Malinowski with reports from Joseph R. LaPlante and Bob Jagolinzer told how "school officials yesterday defended their decision to allow a teenage boy who is suffering from AIDS to attend classes at Case Junior High School." The article went on to say that McCarthy was "considering having the boy's doctor, Peter Smith of Providence, or other medical experts speak to parents at the school. A decision, he said, should be made by today."

The account talked about the 625 students attending the junior high and how the AIDS-stricken teenager had been attending the school since classes began, August 27. The case appeared to be the first in the nation in which a child with AIDS had knowingly been allowed to remain in a public school system. (My principal, Sister Martha Mulligan, had said right along that if Swansea didn't allow Mark to go to school, he could attend St. John's.)

The story went on to tell how "several parents had kept their children home from school." Many were frightened by the news. Principal Harold Devine, however, said he "was aware of only two students who did not attend school because of the boy with AIDS." Mr. Devine gave advice to "call your pediatrician."

Quoting the *Journal*, "Most teachers would not discuss the case, but Marlene Cabral said she supported McCarthy's decision. 'There are varied opinions among teachers,' she said. 'No child asked me questions today.'"

The *Journal* article continued, "Reaction among students was mixed. Eighth-grader Tina Gillotti said she thinks the boy is courageous. The issue, she said, was discussed in her social studies class. 'We talked about his right to learn in our school,' she said. Michael Connors, 13, however, said he was worried about 'the chance of getting it.' Earlier yesterday, all but one of seven parents interviewed as they dropped off their children at school said they supported the district's decision to allow the teenager to attend. 'I definitely think it was the right decision,' said Richard Bourgeois, who has a daughter at the school. 'I'm sure they have taken precautions. I think the boy has rights like everyone else, and has a right to an education.' And Kathy Ryan, a teacher with two children attending the school, said: 'I support the decision as a parent and as a teacher. I think the decision to allow him to attend school is both morally correct and courageous.'"

And how did Mark feel about all this publicity? He liked it and said he always wanted to be famous. The thing that struck him as funny was that some people were afraid to be with him. "When did I first come down with AIDS?" he would ask. "I might have had this in my system for years and it just came out and showed itself in June. I've been going to school with some of these kids since kindergarten." And Mark was right! There is no definite time that we can pinpoint. Some of his classmates could have been near him years ago and he could have had AIDS then. In fact, in 1984 Mark was very, very sick. He had a bad cold the whole month of January and part of February, too. On March 1, he had a strep throat, fever, and an enlarged spleen. When we went to the doctors for a recheck on the 14th, he still had a strep throat, fever, enlarged spleen, swollen glands, and a low blood count. But a mono test was negative. On the 28th he visited Fall River Pediatrics again with an ear infection. His throat had cleared up, but he still had swollen glands, fever, and enlarged spleen.

On April 7, we were back at Pediatrics because he wasn't feeling well. Mark had developed a rash on his face and hands that later spread to his chest, arms, legs, and back. He had another mono test which proved negative, but his blood counts were still low.

Two days later we were back at Pediatrics. We had now seen Dr. Delaney, Dr. Koterbay, and Dr. Penn. Dr. Penn decided to make an appointment at Rhode Island Hospital because Mark's neck was bothering him more and more. It was very stiff. His stomach area was also tender when touched. He still had a fever and didn't have his appetite.

On April 11 we saw Dr. Smith at Rhode Island Hospital. He told us that it wasn't what we were thinking. I wasn't thinking anything, but I guess Dale had suspicions back then in 1984 that Mark had AIDS.

By April 13 Mark was no better and now his back was aching, too. Dr. Smith had put him on dicloxacillan and Tylenol with codeine.

In the middle of the night on April 14 Mark woke up in pain. He needed the Tylenol with codeine every four hours to stay comfortable.

By the 15th, he was getting a little better. The 16th was his best day yet. By the 17th, he was completely off the Tylenol and getting his appetite back. Later that month he was able to go back to school and resume his Little League. What did he have? Was it an AIDS-related virus? I guess we'll never know. Mark was fine after that until May of 1985 when he became sick. So, yes, Mark, it was funny that some people were trying to avoid you.

The *Boston Globe* ran another story about Mark and a survey asking the question, "Should children with AIDS be allowed to attend public schools?" Most people responded favorably to the question. Here are a few of the comments:

Michael Krigman, 27, of Cambridge: "I think so because the only way they can catch it is through sexual contact, and kids 12 or 13, at that age they really don't have close sexual contact. The little kids, it's not their fault they catch it, that they're hemophiliacs and get it through blood transfusions. . . . These kids are already going through enough, they should be allowed to go to school with the rest of the kids."

Nancy Weir, mother of a 15-year-old daughter: "I think they definitely should be allowed to attend school. This poor kid, it isn't his fault. These kids shouldn't be treated as outcasts. The way they get AIDS, they had no control. It's very sad. The only way other kids can get it is through sexual contact or dirty needles—none of which they should be doing in school anyhow."

Saroj Joshi, 48, of Dedham: "I think they should be because it's not contagious. As long as parents and children are told so the parents can tell their children what the disease is all about and about ways they should refrain from certain types of contact with a child with AIDS."

Annette Andrutis, 23, of Boston: "They should be allowed to attend school. How many kids are going to have sexual contact in schools? They always have this big deal about kids with diseases, like when kids have herpes, whether they should be let in the classes. . . . I can see how parents worry about rough play, the kids getting cuts and the disease being transmitted that way. But if you watch the kids, I don't think there's a cause for concern."

Jeanne Foy, 22, of Weymouth: "I think that they should be allowed to go to school. Just because they have a disease, they shouldn't be denied the right to have a public or private education. It's not contagious. If you're just sitting next to me in the classroom, I'm not going to get it."

The *Globe* article said that "reaction was mixed in Swansea with some parents defending the decision while others expressed concern that they had not been notified beforehand." Mr. Devine was asked about the two students being withdrawn from class. 'Two students out of 630 is not a hysterical reaction,' he said. 'Quite frankly, I expected more calls.' Devine went on to say that 'Ninety percent of the faculty is solidly behind the decision the school department has made.'

"Several eighth-graders at the junior high school who know the boy and described him as a shy, quiet 'good kid' yesterday supported the decision to keep him in school. 'I think he can come,' said Denise Dudrick, 13. 'Nobody's going to catch it from him.' The students refused to divulge their classmate's name to reporters, saying they did not want to violate his right to privacy."

Friday, the *Boston Herald* carried two stories about Mark written by Gayle Fee. The headlines were: "Pupils rally 'round AIDS Classmate" and "Diseased boy's family stunned by disclosure." Gayle Fee came to our door on Thursday afternoon. We would not speak to her. Later, my sister Jayne spoke to her in our front yard. Here is her report:

> The 13-year-old Swansea boy who is the center of a raging debate over AIDS victims' rights to public education remained in seclusion yesterday as officials, teachers, students, and neighbors debated his case. (Of course the reason Mark wasn't in school was his ankle problem—not the situation.)
>
> The boy's parents declined to comment on the controversy, but an aunt, who would not give her name, said the public announcement about the boy's disease has been "hell for the family." (That was true.)
>
> "They just found out their kid has been handed a death sentence and they're still trying to accept that, then this has to happen," said the aunt. (Jayne said she didn't say this like it was printed.) "They're just not ready for it. It's a shame this had to get out." The boy had been attending school regularly, played baseball in the local Little League this summer and goes to church every Sunday, the aunt said. "He's fine," she said. "The doctors have said he's OK to go to school. The state Public Health Department said it was OK. Even the Centers for Disease Control said it was OK. What more do people want?" The boy's family fears that once the public learns their son's identity it will be impossible for the youth to continue attending school, his aunt said.
>
> Chris Gorman, the mother of an 8th grader said, "I feel very badly for the boy. I'm sure the attention is going to force him to leave school and that's too bad."

Gayle Fee went on to talk about Mr. McCarthy's opinion and other official positions. Then she put quotes of some students in her article:

> Students said the AIDS victim—who did not attend school yesterday—is a good student, an outstanding athlete, and a "great kid, who doesn't deserve this. He's a

pretty good friend of mine," said 13-year-old Adam Pel-letier. "I live near him, play baseball with him, and hang around with him, but I'm not worried about the disease." Eighth-grader Ronnie Parker said teachers yesterday explained to students how the disease is transmitted. "I think they should just leave him alone and let him go to school."

Charles E. Foy of Fall River, Massachusetts, wrote an editorial letter in support of letting Mark in school. In one of his paragraphs he wrote, "Today we find an element of so-called society looking down their noses at such of the nation's citizens that are less fortunate than ourselves. They have the colossal gall to be self-annointed medical scientists, judge and jury over the lives and happiness of innocent invalids."

The clergy of Somerset and Swansea also wrote an editorial letter entitled: "Clergy has message for AIDS victim, family." It was a wonderful letter of support. In part it said, "We want the patient and his family to know that we support them with our continued prayers and stand ready to aid them in tangible ways. Quite apart from the social issues the tragedy raises, we assure the family of our continued concern and solidarity with them as they travel this most difficult pilgrimage. Rev. Alden Burhoe, Rev. William Nash, Rev. David Movsovich, Rev. Paul Whitteberry, Rev. Merrill Emery, and Rev. Leon Tavitian."

I guess news of Swansea spread throughout the country. Friends in Pennsylvania and South Carolina told me the story was in their papers. Friends visiting Washington, D.C., saw it in papers there. The *Delaware County Daily Times* of September 6 had the headline: "AIDS scare rocks school." It had the whole story about Mark and then had these student comments: "'I'm not scared,' said Joseph Sousa, 13, who is in the sixth grade. 'He's just the same thing as a regular kid, except he had problems. Our science teacher said we should treat him just like we did before he had AIDS.' Denise Ondrich, 14, an eighth grader said, 'Everyone is really good friends with him. They say it's not catchy. I know I'm not going to get it.'"

Later, friends told us that Mark's story was in the papers in Japan and England.

On Friday, September 6, the *Fall River Herald-News* had another headline: "School officials back AIDS victim." It was a nice article stating how business was being maintained as usual at the junior high school. It also mentioned a meeting planned for the parents for the following week.

On Saturday, Mark's ankle seemed to be getting worse. We had to rate each bleed on a scale of one to three for mild, moderate, and severe. I marked it down as a #3 severe bleed. He was taking Demerol which seemed to help somewhat.

The Saturday papers had front page stories again about Swansea. A meeting was scheduled for Wednesday at 7 P.M. at Case High School. It would be attended by health professionals, local school officials, and an official from the Massachusetts Department of Education. Dr. Peter Smith, Mark's doctor; Dr. George F. Grady, an epidemiologist in the state Department of Health; and Curtis Hall, regional director of the state Department of Education, would also be on hand.

Mark couldn't go to school the following week because of his ankle. It just wasn't responding to treatment. He had received double treatments Monday through Wednesday, but the ankle didn't get any better. I continued to pick up his homework at the office each morning. Mr. Devine would always have a little chat with me and let me know what was going on with the press and the public. Mark kept up with his work and spent the rest of his days watching TV or working on his baseball cards. He had to walk around on crutches.

3

*"I think it's something I will remember—
that in this one place, on this most
difficult of issues, the voices of emotion
were drowned out by the voices of reason."*

—Mark Patinkin in the
Providence Journal-Bulletin

Wednesday came, the day of the big important meeting. The date was September 11, 1985. Dale's mother knew how nervous we would be so she invited us down for supper. After supper we were planning on driving home when I got a call from my brother Jeff who lives across the street from us. He warned me that the press was all over the street. They had been ringing our doorbell with camera crews all set to roll. Reporters and TV crews were parked in front of our house and down at the corner. We decided that we'd stay at Dale's mother's. Dale didn't want to leave Mark so she decided to stay at her mother's with Mark and Scott. I would have plenty of company at the meeting, however. My mother, my sister and her husband Dale, my brother Jon (my brother Jeff came late), my father-in-law Tony, my brother-in-law Ken and his wife Nancy and a friend of my sister's all went with me. We sat in one row about three-fourths of the way back right in the middle of the auditorium. Dale had asked me please not to say anything. She felt, and I did too, that it would be better if the whole family just listened and didn't say a word. I saw a lot of people I knew from Little League, Cub Scouts, and just from being a Swansea citizen. Some of my good friends were there and friends of my family.

More than 50 journalists showed up to cover the event. All the major television networks had representatives present. These news reporters and photographers were limited to one section in the front of the auditorium, and they were not allowed to ask questions until the parents had finished. Television crews had to take a feed from the one camera allowed in the high school. It is estimated that more than 700 parents showed up for the meeting. I know there weren't too many empty seats.

I think it is important to record here what happened that evening. The following edited account conveys what took place.

Mr. Devine: Good evening. First I'd like to read a very brief statement for the benefit of the press. All members of the press are confined to the area in the front and to the right of the auditorium. Seating has been reserved for this purpose. Photographers are to remain in the same area as the reporters and are to refrain from entering the aisles at any time following the beginning of the meeting.

The purpose of tonight's meeting is to explain to parents all of the reasoning behind the decisions that have been made. It also serves as the proper forum for you, the parent, to raise your concerns to the appropriate authorities. We hope that by the conclusion of this session you will be satisfied with the decisions that have been made and we will be able to concentrate our energies on educating all of the students at Case Junior High School.

This meeting is for parents of children attending Case Junior High School. We have set up additional seating and we have provided for a cable feed in the library. Since all of the seats in the auditorium are not yet full, we will not ask those who are not parents to leave at this time. If it becomes a problem and we have parents who cannot get into the hall, we will then be forced to ask people who are not parents to go into the library.

Tonight's meeting will be divided into two parts. The first part will consist of a presentation from the individuals seated at the table in the front of the hall. Following the formal presentations, parents will have an opportunity to ask questions of the speakers. My role will be to serve as your moderator and to attempt to direct the flow of information in some sort of logical and efficient manner.

Our first presenter is Dr. Peter S. Smith. Dr. Smith is one of the attending physicians of the stricken child. Dr. Smith is the director of the Hemophilia Center of Rhode Island and is an assistant professor of pediatrics at the Brown University School of Medicine. Dr. Smith.

Dr. Smith: Thank you, Mr. Devine. I would also like to thank you and Mr. McCarthy and the authorities for your courage in facing decisions which must have been difficult considering the pressures that existed and for realizing all the while, probably with an inward joy, that you were doing the right thing. My goal in coming here is to explain to you why it is so important to me personally that this child be allowed back into school and why I think it represents absolutely no risk to you at all.

In hemophilia, which is a hereditary illness, it has been regular practice to exclude children that are afflicted with the disease from school on the premise that they actually represent not only a risk to themselves, but a risk to the schools themselves. Schools have always felt responsible for the care of their children and have been reluctant to accept them in their midst simply because they were afraid of some of the trauma that could occur.

After 1965, when cryoprecipitate was discovered and when concentrates were then distilled from the cryoprecipitates, a tremendous bound forward in the treatment of these cases occurred and children, who formerly would bleed frequently and have to go to hospitals and spend countless hours in waiting rooms, were then able to treat themselves and actually interrupt the bleeding episodes before any damage could occur. This was a real revolution in hemophilia care and we saw kids who had been confined to their homes, behind TV sets, children who were ostracized, who had developed no social skills, finally coming back into their normal setting where they would thrive best—and this was the school, the classroom. I saw that step happen when, together with the National Hemophilia Foundation, our legislators initiated the comprehensive care program in Rhode Island. I personally know many children who were entirely confined behind closed doors and who had really lost the joy of life because of that, and these people were now able to come back into the classroom and develop in the normal way.

Now like all good things, there's always a risk which is attendant upon it. And what you need to know about hemophilia is that the product which is used to treat the disease is derived from literally thousands of donors. The plasmas are pooled from these individuals in donor centers which recruit in various ways, sometimes rather questionable ways, and this plasma is literally poured into vats and the plasma is gradually freeze-dried and all the things that need to come from it are brought out. So in one small vial, about that size (Dr. Smith had his fingers about three inches apart), you may actually have had something like 25,000 donors. Now there is no method in the world which is 100% accurate in detecting any kind of antigen, any kind of infectious agent; we know that is the case with hepatitis B, of which Dr. Grady will be speaking, as a model of this type of condition.

A person with hemophilia, over a course of time, is going to be exposed to thousands and thousands of donors and the chances of his then becoming infected, for instance with hepatitis B, are very great indeed. In this particular condition two things are very important. One is the size of the innoculum, in other words, the number of organisms which are actually being infused into you. And hemophiliacs have to take this concentrate derived from thousands of donors, draw it up into a syringe, insert it into their veins, and give it to themselves. So every time they infuse, and that's approximately once a week for the average hemophiliac, they are infusing these substances. That's one thing, the size of the innoculum. The other thing is the body's defense against harm. We speak of that as the immunity of the body. Now briefly, there is something very exciting about the immunity of the body. In spite of exposure to thousands and thousands of foreign proteins and infectious agents, most of us can fend off all kinds of infectious agents. However, some people do not have that ability. And it is thought that we may be actually speaking of a certain subset of people that are more prone to develop certain kinds of infections and certainly this seems to be the case in hemophiliacs. Because we know that although there are at least 20,000 hemophiliacs in this country, less than 1% of these people have actually developed AIDS. So this is to tell you that in the magnificent experiment that we have been able to conduct in hemophiliacs, we have not seen AIDS to be a very major problem in terms of numbers; the primary cause of death in hemophiliacs is still bleeding. And we now know the longevity of hemophiliacs, if you take all of the hemophiliacs, is still pretty much normal.

Now, what do we know about this AIDS agent that is very relevant? We know for one thing that researchers have been unable to isolate it out of the concentrates which were looked at at the Centers for Disease Control, so they must be infinitesimally small amounts. But it's the repetitiveness, the infusion over a longer, longer period of time that seems to be making the difference. So that's telling us something. It's telling us that it's very hard to get AIDS. It's not easy to get AIDS, it's not done by casual contact. What are the other sources of exposure which cause the disease AIDS to manifest itself? It is in other situations where intimate contact with exchange of secretions occur. These are the situations we're talking about: we're talking about repeated sexual intercourse in a variety of ways — and particularly anal intercourse. So this is one of the facts that we need to know.

I have mentioned to you that the reason why I'm here in a way is because I'm an advocate obviously; but the other reason is that the hemophilia community has been able to research this disease probably better than anybody, because we all form a very large network of interrelated hemophilia centers. We all talk with each other, we're all aware of the risks that are about, and we've all been reading about this since the first reports came out in 1981. We've been looking retrospectively at the data and we've been able to look also at families who have been exposed over a longer period of time to our patients with AIDS and we've been able to show that these exposures have not resulted in any case with any clinical manifestations of AIDS, let alone to any conversion of the serum. So, I think that the message that I am bringing and I hope to impart right here is that the risk of catching AIDS in a casual manner, meaning by being around a person with AIDS, being breathed on by a person, shaking hands, is extremely remote, so remote that I would call it less likely than you succumbing to something like an automobile accident, by stepping in front of a car, falling off a bicycle, or falling out the window. That's the type of probabilities we're talking about. And that's why I think that you

can be very proud of yourselves that you may actually represent one of the first communities which knowingly has allowed a victim with AIDS to come into your school.

Mr. Devine: Thank you, Dr. Smith. Our next presenter is Dr.
George F. Grady. Dr. Grady is the assistant commissioner for
the Massachusetts Department of Public Health. He is the
state epidemiologist, the senior physician, scientist, for the
Commonwealth in charge of preventive medicine and disease
control policy. Dr. Grady is the director of the state Laboratory
Institute for the diagnosis of disease of public health impor-
tance. He is a professor of medicine, infectious diseases, at the
Tufts University School of Medicine. He is a consultant to the
AIDS research task forces of the Federal Centers for Disease
Control and the National Institute of Health. He is a member
of the governor's task force and a nationally known researcher
on the causes and prevention of viral diseases. Dr. Grady.

Dr. Grady: Thank you. If you don't mind I'll stand up. I also
consider it an honor and a privilege to be able to come here
tonight. Dr. Smith has told you why he thinks it's in the child's
interest to be able to attend school like any other child and of
the great advances that have been made in the opening up of
a normal world to children, and now adults, with hemophilia.
And he's done a very eloquent job of that, and I'm certainly not
going to repeat it because I think a natural sympathy for and
knowledge of this particular child and his family is what has
allowed this community to, shall we say, suspend judgment,
that is to say, to repress the normal fright instinct at least until
you could get more information, which is the purpose of this
meeting tonight and the purpose of earlier information that's
been given to you.

I'm not going to spend any more time taking the case of the
child who's involved; I'll take a very coldblooded look at the no-
tion of what's good for most of the people. In other words, I
don't want this to be viewed as a liberal, emotional commitment of risk-taking for the sake of one of our own. I submit to
you that there is no risk. If there were a risk, much as I might
identify with the child, I would feel it would be my responsibility to tell you that, and that the rights of the majority should

not be subordinated to the rights of the minority. But under the situation and conditions we're talking about here, I consider the risks zero.

Let's just narrow down what we do know and don't know about AIDS. There are basic researchers now who are unraveling the structure down to the atomic level of the AIDS virus. And not all of that work is unraveled. Nor have the mysteries been completely unraveled as to exactly how it affects the immune system and leads to disease. But, in contrast to that incomplete information, we know a very great deal about how it is transmitted. In fact, we know so much, I think there is an underestimation of just how much we do know. This disease is tracking and recapitulating and following exactly the course of discovery and documentation of transmission patterns that happened about 20 years ago with the disease hepatitis.

I have sort of flashbacks to that disease because, in the early days, I would stand before groups like this talking about risks to hospital employees, and to teachers and others. After a while, it became understood and accepted that, although the virus is present in certain individuals, that is not synonymous with transmissibility. There is really only one way that has stood up in terms of transmission methods for AIDS and that is a blood-to-blood or serum-to-serum type of contact. Now, that's the common denominator, but there's several varieties of that transmission. One would be the need to take a blood concentrate distillate, as Dr. Smith referred to, which, since it comes from thousands of donors, statistically might be infected. That has been the unfortunate lot of many hemophiliacs. The good news, however, that I would hasten to add, is that there are now new techniques for decontaminating or inactivating those products. This should spare that risk for children now being born with hemophilia. That's the good news. So we're dealing with a transitional phenomena here of a certain number of people who unavoidably were exposed before the techniques for taking care of that problem were recognized.

The second variation on the blood-to-blood transmission is that in the past if you needed a blood transfusion, you were dependent on the goodwill, the honesty, accuracy of the blood donor in giving a complete health history, to the extent that they knew it, that they were not likely to be a carrier of a diseased particle. But tests have been developed and are now in place and every single unit of blood being donated is being screened. And the only peculiarity is that during this transitional period, it has been discovered that some people who transfused as long as a couple of years earlier, may then after a long delay show the AIDS disease. But that's extremely rare, perhaps one in 500,000 transfusions. You would have to be very unlucky to be that individual. And furthermore, that's past tense, that period is over. The screening is now eliminating that problem in the blood transfusion situation. The testing is probably 95–99% successful. I shouldn't say eliminating, nothing is ever quite perfect, but it's largely eliminated.

The third variation would be people, who for various reasons of escapism or whatever, experiment with injectable drugs, so-called recreational drugs. If those needles are contaminated with small amounts of blood, the virus particles that cause this family of diseases can be present in the blood, contaminating the needles or syringes, and can transfer the infection from person to person. That's just one more reason why we have to really bear down on trying to educate our kids that it's not funny to deal with drugs. If the purpose is self-destruction, one might get there in more ways than you would anticipate. So all those have the common denominator of blood-to-blood.

What about sexual contact? In fact, it's looking more and more like not just any sexual contact, even with an infected person, will transmit AIDS, it probably has to take place across somewhat raw or inflamed surfaces. So there is some actual serum or blood-to-blood exchange. The mystery is beginning to disappear from the disease. Not handshakes, not toilet seats, not sneezing, not coughing, not water coolers will convey the disease, nor just the presence in a donor person who has it, but a very complicated sequence of events has to take place. There has to be a lot of virus in the initiating person, there has to be an opening for it to get out, it has to match up in turn with an opening, find its way through the body of the recipient, who in addition has to be especially susceptible as Dr. Smith said. If AIDS were anything like, as communicable as, other childhood diseases that you might otherwise think about, like measles or whatever, everyone in this audience would have been infected by now. But it is not a casually transmitted disease. So under the circumstances that I understand to exist here and which were discussed with Superintendent McCarthy, we have a highly motivated child, who is intelligent, does not want in any way to let his own personal health or hygiene lapse, is not going to be bleeding all over people, and is simply not a threat sitting in the next seat. Those are the circumstances under which by definition I consider the risk zero.

When consulted about whether one should tack a notice on the door or something of that sort and say we have this situation, I share the responsibility for advising against it for the simple reason that the mystery factor and fright factor is so great that that's tantamount to saying that no one can go to school. This is not a small crowd here and if you can imagine having the media like this here daily, as has happened in other cities, you might as well say the judgment has already been made, we don't care what you doctors and scientists think, we're frightened, there should be no school, or there should not be this child. On the other hand, I do not feel that anyone who is afraid or initially afraid before they hear this information should have to apologize for their fear or anxiety. It's impossible with the media barrage we've had not to have these concerns. And that's why I do consider it a privilege to come here and answer your questions. I've left my work number and even my home number for any particular parents who've been concerned to call me directly and have been pleased that I've been able to talk at length to several people who, I'm sure, are here in the audience tonight, and answer their specific concerns. But we do know a lot about this disease and we find that it's tracking exactly like other diseases with which we've had even more experience and there is no mystery in its transmission pattern. And so that is the basis on which I speak to you tonight and I'll be glad to answer questions later when the session is appropriate. Thank you.

Mr. Devine: Our next speaker is Mr. Curtis Hall. Mr. Hall is the director of the Southeast Region Center for the State Department of Education and as such is the highest ranking state educational official in this area. Mr. Hall.

Mr. Hall: Thank you. My role tonight is perhaps a little different because I bring to you not knowledge of the medical profession, but knowledge of what the Department of Education expects when a medical decision has been made.

On September 6, the commissioner for Public Health and the commissioner of Education issued publicly a joint statement relative to AIDS. As a person in public education for 34 years, I looked at that statement and I said "strike the word 'AIDS'" and I find that the existence of that policy has been there forever. In fact, it has its basis in law, chapter 76, section 1, which is that section of the law pertaining to compulsory education. Each and every one of us in this audience is aware of the fact that when one attends school, they may be relieved of their responsibility to attend school upon medical excuse. The medical profession has always been looked to by the education profession to make judgments as to the appropriateness of a particular child's attendance or non-attendance. And that appropriateness is in two parts. One, is it safe for the child, in terms of that individual child, to attend in a public school setting? Two, is it safe and appropriate for that child to attend in a public school setting, relative to the other children surrounding that child? That decision has been made by appropriate medical persons. It is the opinion of the Department of Education, the commissioner, and the Board of Education that I represent, that the decision having been made, that the Swansea Public Schools have appropriately interpreted and carried out the mandates for a compulsory education. And, in fact, they have done those things which we would assume would be done in any community in the Commonwealth of Massachusetts. I join my colleagues on the panel in saying that, even though you bring questions to this room, this town, this community, must stand proud and I'm just pleased and proud to have the opportunity to come and talk to a community where you have brought your questions into the open, you have called persons in the proper and appropriate manner and, in fact, you have respected the regulation that I think is appropriate in this case — that is, the right of this discussion to go forth protecting the confidentiality of individuals involved. Our regulations, both state and federal, require that and I just think it's a tremendous tribute to the respect that you bring to each other and to your leadership and to the students in this community and that you're able to acknowledge it. I'm here for any questions on that aspect of the situation.

Mr. Devine: John E. McCarthy is the superintendent of schools in Swansea. Superintendent McCarthy will explain to you the basis for the decisions that have been made.

Mr. McCarthy: Thank you, Mr. Devine. As your school superintendent, it was my responsibility, when I first learned that a child had been diagnosed as having acquired immune deficiency syndrome, to approach the proper authorities and look for guidance. I began by contacting the Centers for Disease Control in Atlanta, the State Department of Education, the State Department of Public Health, and I began to learn how it was that one would determine whether or not such a child presented a risk to others. During my investigation it became very clear to me from all the experts that, indeed, there was no public risk. At that point in time, the next decision that I had to make was how to best handle this situation. The guidelines that have been published by the proper agencies that deal with these matters state quite emphatically that only those persons with an absolute need to know in the educational and public health field are to receive this information. Indeed, the public guidelines also say the initial responsibility for reporting this matter rests with the child's attending physician. The attending physician is to report this matter to public health officials on the state level and to the school superintendent. It then becomes the responsibility of the school superintendent to identify those persons with this need to know. The guidelines spell out that such persons are the school principal, the school nurse, and teacher. Since this was a secondary school situation we were dealing with, the term "teacher" applied to many persons, because in secondary schools there are several teachers who are assigned programs to teach all the children.

We made those people with an absolute need to know informed, in the best manner that we could. Subsequent to that, when the need to know seemed to extend to the entire school staff, we also had a briefing with the entire school staff. We had planned at a future time to also carry out recommendations that are included in these guidelines to approach the public on an informational and educational basis. Unfortunately, the time span required to establish such an educational program did not allow us to do this. By the stories that broke in the news media, we were then required to proceed with the particular meeting that we are having here this evening. And of all the questions that have been asked of me concerning procedures, the one question that comes up over and over again is "Why didn't you tell us?" And the reason I didn't tell you is because all throughout this procedure I have done exactly as I am supposed to do; I followed the guidelines to the letter. Hopefully your concerns and questions will be answered here this evening. It is my opinion that we have the best experts in the field available to answer your questions. Thank you. (applause)

Mr. Devine: At this time it would be appropriate for you, the parents, to ask questions of our guests. For the purpose of order and efficiency, the following procedures will be in effect: 1) Please do not attempt to speak until you have been recognized by me and until you have received a microphone. We have microphones on both sides of the auditorium. Once you are recognized, please stand, and a microphone will be brought to you. Upon being recognized and receiving the microphone, kindly state your name and address. As was mentioned at the outset, the purpose of this meeting is to hold the kind of discussion that is taking place now with the parents of the children attending Case Junior High School. This discussion is confined to the parents of students attending Case Junior High School. Every speaker has the right to a point of view. Any demonstration of approval or disapproval for any point of view expressed will only delay our proceedings. I would ask that all questions be asked through me. When you state your question, if you would be kind enough to tell me which guest you would like to respond to your question, I will direct the question to the appropriate guest. We hope that these procedures will ensure a logical exchange of information. I would mention at this time that you have already heard the phrase "we're following the guidelines," the school department has reproduced 300 copies of the complete guidelines which were put out just this past week by the Massachusetts State Department of Education. These will be made available to you at the conclusion of this evening's meeting. At this time it would be appropriate to address questions to our panelists. Sir.

Speaker: My question is, I guess, to Mr. McCarthy.

Mr. Devine: Excuse me, would you identify yourself and state your address please? [In the interest of privacy, this account will omit last names and addresses.]

Speaker: My name is Dennis B———. My daughter's in eighth grade. In light of the medical profession, excuse me if I'm not in awe of it, I think everyone here has had some sort of a problem with them. There's been drugs that have come out that really hasn't been exactly what they thought it was going to be and that sort of thing. But I'm not here to chastise the medical profession. My question is, with this in mind, why couldn't we have waited six months or a year to get maybe more information for the simple reason, if we're wrong, what are we exposing our children to? If we're right, in putting it off for six months, what is the worst that could possibly happen? But what is the worst that could possibly happen if we're wrong?

Mr. Devine: Thank you. *(interrupted by applause)* Again, before directing that question to Mr. McCarthy, I would ask your cooperation in permitting the exchange of information to proceed freely without demonstration. It will certainly speed things up and make for a much more informative evening. Thank you. Mr. McCarthy.

Mr. McCarthy: Yes, Mr. B———, to reply to your question. Based on what I consider a rather thorough investigation that I conducted during the time that I investigated this matter and talked to the authorities, I saw no need to twice jeopardize a victim who had already been given, if I can say, a poor deal in life. I didn't see what was to be gained by waiting six months, and I didn't see any need for socially isolating a youngster and adding to a situation that was already very difficult to live with. I saw no need in that. And I thought the best advantage for this child, since there was no risk to anyone else, was to have that child working in a classroom setting with other children where he belonged and where he had been functioning—throughout the entire summer playing Little League baseball—being with his classmates. *(applause)*

Mr. Devine: Further questions? Over here on the aisle, please.

Dr. Grady: Mr. Devine, could I respond further to the question, please? I think it's fair to say doctors don't know everything. That's one of my favorite phrases. And I also think that you always know a little bit more if you wait longer than if you don't wait. But this is not the zero point in examining this question. Perhaps I'm guilty of not stressing in my presentation that there has never been a case of child-to-child transmission of this disease. And this disease has been with us for at least five years—maybe more—so what you're really saying is why not wait five years and six months instead of five years. In other words, this is not the zero point. . . . I'm not diminishing the value that additional time may add something, but we're getting out pretty far in the level of knowledge so that's really my interpretation of the question.

Mr. Devine: Thank you, Doctor. Yes, ma'am.

Speaker: Janet C———. In all the cases that have been diagnosed as AIDS, what I'd like to know is how many of the siblings or parents have they done research on to see if they've contracted this disease?

Mr. Devine: Dr. Smith?

Dr. Smith: I was mentioning to you what an ideal situation it was in the hemophilia population because they have been basically captive, unfortunately, because of their disease and they've always required close medical attention. In data which will soon be published, in more than 100 families who have specifically been investigated, there has been no evidence of any other sibling and families sero-converting, in other words, showing any markers of the disease in the blood. And believe me, this is being around all the time, being at the same table, eating out of the same dishes, being around somebody who bleeds, so the risk has been very low and, again, this has been an unwanted biological experiment, but we do know those facts.

Mr. Devine: Thank you, further questions? Yes, ma'am.

Speaker: My question is for Dr. Grady.

Mr. Devine: Could you identify yourself, please?

Speaker: I'm Mary Anne G———. I have a daughter in the sixth grade. You said that certain types of individuals were more susceptible to the disease, I guess you mean that they cannot fight off the disease. Am I correct on that before I go on with my question? They don't have the ability as well, certain types of individuals do not have the ability to fight off the disease as well as perhaps other people? Do you feel that there are any certain types of chronically ill children that are susceptible, other than hemophiliacs, to the AIDS or hepatitis B virus?

Mr. Devine: Thank you, Mrs. G———. Dr. Grady?

Dr. Grady: Well, I think that maybe it was Dr. Smith who pointed out that not everyone exposed develops the classical form of AIDS and to further that again, for the sake of time, maybe I should have explained a little bit more about what AIDS is. It's not a disease at all like chicken pox or measles, or whatever. People often say to me, how much fever do you get with AIDS, or what does the rash of AIDS look like? The question itself shows that there is not an understanding of what's happening here. What happens is that there is a slow and gradual involvement, based on the virus that causes AIDS, that weakens the total body resistance, so that germs that are in the air here in this auditorium that are very mild germs and to which we all have the great capacity to resist, cannot be resisted by a person with AIDS. So the diagnosis is not made instantly, but what happens is that a child or adult comes back to a hospital or a doctor, either once with a very unusual infection by a germ that normally could not affect a normal person, or they come back several times with a series of odd infections. And so it's only then, often quite late, that one recognizes, in retrospect, that this might have been an AIDS infection.

Now there are many other conditions which can weaken a person's natural immunity. Some children are born with those conditions; there may be a variety of other conditions, but it's not a condition that I personally think would make them in any way vulnerable, or more vulnerable to the AIDS virus. Because what we're really talking about here is a determination based on opportunity from massive transfer of blood and blood-containing products. And the whole basis of my statement is that under the circumstances of the state policy, it does not say that all children with AIDS should go to school automatically, or that they should not. It says, and I will repeat, that children who are of normal motivation, normal psychological make-up, are well enough in the eyes of their physician to be able to handle themselves well in school, do not have open, weeping sores, and are not the kind of child who would go and bite someone and therefore create the capacity to transfer this virus—under all those conditions, that this is a safe and zero-risk situation. . . . In short, I don't know of any children who are well enough to go to school who have any special reason to fear the non-transfer that I'm talking about. I mean, to me, I just don't see the connection.

Mr. Devine: Further questions? Let me go toward the back. Yes, sir, on the aisle.

Speaker: OK, I'm Lenny C———. We've been through hell for about a week and a half to two weeks. After the kids all went to school, that's when the parents were notified of this. I'm talking to all the parents, they must have went through hell, too. We got on the phone, we called Atlanta, Georgia. We called all over. I must have made about $100 worth of phone calls. What you gentlemen are saying here tonight, we've heard the same thing, but they didn't give us any definite answer, they said like this, there's a possibility that you can get this by body sweat from the youngster that's in school. I asked them again, I said, is that a possibility my kid would not get it? He could get it! Now another question is, now we've heard our own doctors, our doctors, the kid's doctors said the same thing. Now on TV we heard these doctors, on NBC, this morning, yesterday morning, and the host of the show asked them, "Is it a possibility that a kid could go to school without getting this?" They would not guarantee it. We've got kids, all of us, coming to this school; when they leave the house, we expect them to be safe—nothing's safe really—but you ain't gonna leave a kid go around with a match with a gallon of gas and this is what it looks like to me. Because no one, everybody knows what AIDS are, can be, but nobody has a cure for and nobody can control it.

Now, another point, the parents were notified of this two weeks after the kid went to school. Now I think the parents should have been notified before school started. (*applause*) Gentlemen, Mr. McCarthy down there, I got four sons, one of them goes down to 18 months old, I got to live with it. I don't know how you other people in the audience feel, but this is a sickness that there's no comeback like the flu and 10 days, get a shot, go back to school. Your kids live with this and they die with it. Now another thing is, if this wasn't brought out to the press, all of you here, would you know about it? (*Some say "no."*) I wonder, Mr. McCarthy, answer that one please.

Mr. Devine: Excuse me, Mr. C———, if you're going to ask a question, please ask the question.

Speaker: I'm asking it, I'm talking about the lives of my sons and everybody else's sons and daughters in this room.

Mr. Devine: Mr. C———, I'm sure that everyone else will have an opportunity to make whatever points they wish to make.

Speaker: That's right and I'm here tonight to find out because this is life or death, sir! (*some applause*) Who is to say that my son or my daughter is all right to come to school, knowing that this could be a deadly disease? And they sit down there saying that my son could go out to war and die, well, it's not so. Why didn't the gentleman down there that made the good statement, why didn't they wait another six months? The doctor says, why don't you wait another five years and six months? My son could have died by then, my other son could have died by then, your daughter could have died by then! No! Thank you, Mr. McCarthy, answer that one though!

Mr. Devine: Are there any further questions? (*some talking in auditorium*) Let's go over to this side, yes, ma'am. (*some talking in auditorium*) Excuse me, we'll hold that, we'll hold that. Number one, I heard a speech, I didn't really hear a question. (*more talking*) And I would hope, excuse me, no one is going to try and hide anything. However, (*more talking*) if we don't attempt to maintain some sort of civil order, we're never going to get any communication at all during this meeting. So Mr. C———, if you would like to ask Mr. McCarthy a question, please do. (*Audience is calling out—"He did!"*)

Dr. Smith: Can I help out on that?

Mr. Devine: Dr. Smith.

Dr. Smith: Mr. C———, let me explain what happened. (*Mr. C——— is saying something without a mike.*) Are you listening? (*Mr. C———: Yes.*) All right. (*Mr. C———: I'm all ears.*) OK. When I found out this boy, who was treated magnificently in a Fall River hospital, had had AIDS, and that I would be taking care of him, I was very aware of the fact that I would have to bring this to the attention of the proper authorities before allowing him to go to school. Before I went on vacation, shortly after the boy was released from the hospital, I asked my secretary to set up a time with Mr. Devine and the appropriate individuals so that we could discuss that. And so I have to say that I bear the responsibility for going on vacation because I went away for two weeks, and I didn't come back until the last day before that Monday. So the meeting in which I could sit down together with my collaborators from the Hemophilia Center, Nancy Keyes and Debbie DeMaio, who are sitting right over here, could take place one day before the boy was to enter school. It was not a deliberate obfuscation of what happened, nor an attempt to sneak the boy into the school without you knowing anything. And I must say, I must take the blame for not getting in touch with him sooner.

Speaker: [*speaking without a mike and hard to hear him clearly*] Now the boy played baseball with my son. He was on the Giants and my son was on the Red Sox. Now they knew this in July or June when the All-Star team came up. That boy did not play baseball after July or June because he came down with a sickness and was in the hospital. [Actually, Mark did go back and play for a couple of games.]

Mr. Devine: Mr. McCarthy, would you like to respond to Mr. C——?

Mr. McCarthy: Yes, I certainly would. Mr. C——, you have four children, I have six. I would share the same concern that you do and I called the proper authorities, I made that statement up front, I got the information. Apparently, your understanding of the information is a little bit different than mine, but the authorities who are in a position to tell me what we should do said there was absolutely no risk, as these gentlemen have said up here tonight. (*Mr. C—— is saying something.*) Will you please give me a chance to talk now! Thank you. Further, as far as following the guidelines as to what I am supposed to do, I repeated before, I informed only those with an absolute need to know. Apparently, from your statements, you happened to know more than I did—early on. But as far as I'm concerned, I did the absolute right thing. I followed the guidelines, I did exactly as I was supposed to do. Mentioning your four children, perhaps today we are dealing with this particular issue, with this particular child. Five months, six months from now, I could be dealing with another issue with one of your children, and I hope that you would feel that I would be as fair to him as I am trying to be with this other situation. *(loud and long applause)*

Speaker: *(He continued to talk without the mike.)* And who the heck gives you the right without telling us?

Mr. McCarthy: The right to decide who attends school or who does not attend school belongs to the Department of Public Health and the Department of Education. They're the people who make that decision. If I let everybody decide who's going to school and who's not going to go to school based on fear and hysteria, or any other reason, I'm not going to be fair to the individual children and their right to attend school. *(loud and long applause)*

Mr. Devine: Thank you, Mr. C———. I would once again appeal to the audience, tonight's meeting is meant to be informational, not confrontational! I hope that we can walk the line, I hope that we can maintain the spirit of the free flow and dissemination of information without attempting to precipitate any confrontations. We're all on the same side. I had recognized the young lady over here, do you still wish to speak, ma'am?

Speaker: I'm Jean I———. I'm going to ask the two doctors this question. Is the virus spread through body fluids?

Mr. Devine: Is the virus spread through body fluids? Is that your question? Dr. Smith?

Dr. Smith: The virus is carried in tears, saliva, a. . . .

Speaker: Urine?

Dr. Smith: Not the urine, feces. But I think the important thing and the link that is probably lacking here is that it's an incredibly fastidious virus. In other words, the virus is around us all the time. But it takes intimate contact, in other words, blood-born contact, in order actually for the virus to do things. We're bathed in viruses every day yet we don't get them.

Speaker: Yes, we're bathed in viruses every day but it isn't a deadly virus. We die with AIDS. We do not live. And I don't think that we should take a chance with our children. If we love them, we won't take a chance. *(some slight applause)* These people here are brainwashing us. To tell us to send our children to school, when they contract it, it's your problem *(speaking to the parents)* and you did it, not them *(pointing to the panel)*.

When your children are dying (*moans from the audience*), they don't know nothing about AIDS. Nobody's positive of AIDS.

Mr. Devine: Thank you. Are there any further questions?

Speaker: I'm not finished.

Mr. Devine: Do you have another question?

Speaker: Are you familiar with Dr. Wiseman from the UCLA AIDS study clinic?

Dr. Smith: I'm not, but I think Dr. Grady is.

Speaker: Well, he said it's transmitted by the body fluids which you just said; the virus, it is present in saliva.

Dr. Grady: May I respond, unless you have another question?

Speaker: Kids spit. Thank you.

Mr. Devine: Thank you, Dr. Grady.

Dr. Grady: Let me answer the question as best I can. I said before that the most common mistake in understanding the difference between a germ's presence and a germ's transmission is being brought out with AIDS. I think some of the newspaper reporters have properly criticized doctors for saying that on Monday they can't wait to publish the latest study that shows it is found in ear wax, but then on Wednesday they say, but don't worry, it's not a problem. So I don't blame you for being frightened and confused about this. The fact of the matter is that the actual evidence of transmission still is limited after many, many years to blood and serum products. And there are many viruses that have been found in tears or saliva, or whatever, but there's no evidence of that type of transmission. And, in fact, not even the most frightened advocates that I'm aware of have ever come up with one shred of evidence that it is present in sweat. The official opinion of the same people you are quoting is summarized in this report of which extra copies are here, and it goes out of its way to say that it is not transmitted by sweat or these superficial body fluids that you are talking about. This is very clearly the official opinion of the people that are being quoted here tonight . . . . and it does not say what you are hearing being attributed to them. So, I do not believe that sweat is an issue. There have been, under experimental conditions, isolations from tears and from saliva, yes, but there has been no evidence that these play any role in the actual transmission for the reasons that I gave you. Not present in stool, not present in urine, that's it.

Mr. Devine: Further questions? Let's go right to the middle. I see a young lady with her hand in the air. Please stand.

Speaker: My name is Ellen F———. I have eight children, one of which attends the junior high school. First of all, it's neither here nor there as far as I'm concerned whether we should have known it, or we don't know it, we know it now and we're here to learn about it. I have a question to the good doctors, Dr. Smith and Dr. Grady. You have children. Being in the situation we're in, would you hesitate to send your children to school?

Dr. Smith: Thank you for the question. I wouldn't have the slightest hesitation. And it's not because I want to make a martyr out of my child, it's just that we have enough knowledge right now about how this disease is being transmitted to know that it's perfectly safe.

Mr. Devine: Dr. Grady.

Dr. Grady: Yes, thank you, first of all, it's not just to prove a point or to be dramatic about it, but I do believe that people should practice what they preach. I have mentioned that I do have children, I do have children in public school. In fact, I have a boy exactly the same age as this child. . . . In this business, you don't have credibility unless you practice what you preach. And it's quite likely that within a matter of time I will have a chance to prove that point. There are very few children with AIDS, less than 1 or 2% of the total cases are children, but they do tend to occur, more likely, in the more highly populated areas. I live near Boston, so statistically, I may have a chance to prove that point. And I have, in fact, discussed it with my children, and I have said, "Look, you've read a lot about this, aren't you afraid?" And their answer to me was, "Look, we know that you love us, we know you wouldn't want any harm to come to us, and we know that you spent your life looking at this, and you believe this is not a problem—that's good enough for us." That's their answer. [*some applause*]

Mr. Devine: The lady who just stood up in front of Mrs. F———.

Speaker: My name is Terry F———. I've got two children, one in sixth grade and one in eighth grade. I've got a lot of things to say, but I'm not going to start right now. I do think that whoever is responsible for keeping this from us ought to be brought to, brought charges against, or whatever. I also want to know if we can start a petition to either keep the kid away from our children, out of the schools (*the audience moans*), or if the town will pay for our children's education in Somerset, or whatever.

Mr. Devine: Mr. McCarthy?

Mr. McCarthy: Well, if I understand the question, she wants to know if she can bring charges against me, is that the question? (*laughter-applause*) The first question?

Mr. Devine: That's it.

Mr. McCarthy: Guess so, if that's how you feel. (*laughter*) The second question, would the school department pay the tuition of children going to another school system? The answer is no.

Speaker: That's just a part of my question. I want to know if there is a way we can get this child away from my children? That was my question and to see if the town would pay tuition.

Mr. Devine: Thank you, Mrs. F———. Mr. McCarthy.

Mr. McCarthy: Well, I answered the second part of it, the first part of it, regarding the petition, I'll go over the position I made originally, that Mr. Hall from the Department of Education made. What I'm doing is following the regulations that were laid down by the State Department of Education, and also following the directives of the people in public health who make the decision as to whether or not a child attends school. If we take a look at this issue, and if we say we will let public opinion decide who goes and who doesn't go, what happens when the next serious disease comes up? Do we do the same thing there? Do we make a decision based on public opinion? Somebody has to make the call. In the case of a health issue, it's the Department of Public Health, it's Dr. Grady's job. In the case of attendance, it's Mr. Hall and the Department of Education. I follow those directives and it's the only way we can keep some semblance of continuity and sense to this whole business.

Mr. Devine: Let's go over here to the right to the young lady against the wall with the reddish dress.

Speaker: My name is Susan Travers [I use her full name because she later did a great deal for our family by founding a group called the "Friends of Mark."] and I have a son in the sixth grade. There are some areas in the United States that are more heavily populated where AIDS tends to show up more. And I haven't noticed them closing down gyms for people who are contaminated. They still go to gyms, they still go into super-markets, they still go into churches, and hospitals, and we are not seeing any huge outbreaks. I feel that these parents and this child are being punished because they did come forward with this. And I think in anything with our children we take risks; putting them on a school bus, sending them out, today putting them in day care—there's been all kinds of things about what's happening in day care—and yet we send our children out to it every single day. I think that in anything in life, there are risks. And I think we have to support each other. Nobody wants to see anybody's child get sick.

I have to put myself in those parents' place and say to myself if it were me, what would I want? I don't want people to be afraid, yet, I'd have to also think about the child that I have. And my son told me last night that it's the quality of the life that we live here that's great. And you have to think about that, too. And I just think they're being penalized because they're be-ing honest and open. And as far as not knowing, it doesn't make a difference. It doesn't make a difference if we knew six months ago or today, it's not going to go away and we have to deal with it. And we can't not send our children to school and we can't stop this child from being educated. He has a right to that education. *(loud and long applause)*

Mr. Devine: Thank you, Mrs. Travers. Young lady about two-thirds of the way back in the middle section. Yes, ma'am.

Speaker: Yes, I'm Chris F———. I have three boys at the school. I would like to know if there's going to be any informa-tion given to the kids now that we've had this meeting. We made a lot of children panic over something that they don't know about.

Mr. Devine: Let me address that, Mrs. F———. The policy of the school regarding this particular issue has been to deal with it directly with the children as the need arises and this is what has been happening. One of the barometers that I've attempted to use has been cases of concern. If the child is con-cerned, if the child is worried about something, often he or she will seek out our guidance counselor. At this time, no children at Case Junior High School have sought this particular kind of counseling. The teachers are dealing with the issues as they arise within the intimate confines of the classroom. We feel that is the best way to handle the situation. We decided right on against going to large group assemblies, attempting to bring people in to speak to large groups of children. We felt that that would create the type of atmosphere that could lead to emotional kinds of reactions that wouldn't be healthy for the kids. So we're attempting to deal with it during this particular phase, on a need-to-know basis. As the situations arise in the classroom, they're being handled immediately by the teachers. The teachers are also disseminating a sufficient amount of information in order to satisfy the natural curiosity of the children without attempting to inundate them with facts and figures—most of which they wouldn't really care about. Does that answer your question?

Speaker: Yes.

Mr. Devine: Thank you. The young lady that just stood up over here a minute ago.

Speaker: My name is Jody Donnelly. [I use her last name because she is a friend and neighbor who lives on the next street from us.] I have five children. And what you parents are all asking for is a guarantee. You can't even guarantee your next breath that you're going to breathe, only God can do that. But what I want to tell you all is my youngest son, who, if you knew my husband, walks on water as far as he is concerned, is best friends with this afflicted boy's brother. My son has been in their home and I have known about this boy's disease since he came down with it during the summer—I've been aware of it. I have not kept my son from their home. He was over there yesterday, and the boy has been over to my home. If I thought my son was in jeopardy, and I'm in the medical profession myself, I would certainly not put my beloved child in that type of situation where I feel I would be endangering his life. I feel no threat to my son or my other children. And I think the Swansea school system should be commended for their stand and you parents should be proud of your town that they have taken this stand and they have been the first town to do so. And I think it's a proud thing for them to take this stand and I commend everyone. (*loud and long applause*) Put yourself in this family's situation. Have a little bit of compassion for this family and this boy. This is what they need, they need your support, not criticism. (*applause*)

Mr. Devine: Thank you, Mrs. Donnelly. Further questions? Let me go over this way right against the wall.

Speaker: Thank you. My name is Celeste R———. I have one daughter in Case Junior High School. I'd like to pose a question that addresses itself to the future, looking positively on the idea that the child will stay in school and that we'll all support him. I think some of our fears are that we know that AIDS ultimately leads to death. I'd like one of the doctors to maybe walk us through the next year with the progression of the illness of this child so we can have a little bit better understanding. And the second part of my question is, could you tell us from the school department, how you're going to monitor this boy? Because your statement to us now is that he's fine, he can attend school and that's good. However, when he doesn't, or if he doesn't continue to stay in this present state, who will monitor this situation and how will we become aware as parents so we can know what's going on in the school? . . . Because when you talk about death, you worry about that like maybe tomorrow or something, so can we address that please?

Mr. Devine: Thank you. Yes, Dr. Smith.

Dr. Smith: Thank you, very good question. I believe I'm the appropriate person to address that because I probably spend most of my time treating children with cancer. . . .

First of all, I'd like to state that in a field like oncology, or in a field that deals with life-threatening illnesses like AIDS, there's an awful lot of uncertainty there. And therefore, we physicians who are specialized in that kind of disorder, do not go into it thinking that it's a lost cause—that the person is going to be the loser. We approach it realizing that this has been the natural history of medicine, that we may actually witness as time goes, a very hopeful treatment that will come along which will reverse the change. So that's one thing, I think, that to say that 50% of the people who have AIDS have succumbed to AIDS is not implying that the other 50% are also going to die. So the natural history of the survivor of AIDS is not yet known. And believe me, there will be survivors of AIDS. Just as there have been survivors of many other infectious diseases.

We know that with these infectious diseases there is such a thing as dying from them, there's such a thing as having moderate problems from them, and there's such a thing as being a carrier. And in the AIDS situation we now know that there are actually people who carry the virus. That has been demonstrated in a small number of cases that have been closely studied of those who carry the virus but have absolutely no effect from it. So this may very well show us that in the future, those who survive AIDS initially may actually have long term survival.

Now let me take this back down to the basic biology of AIDS. AIDS is a condition in which the virus infects particular types of cells that flow in the blood and these cells are responsible for fighting off foreign stuff; anything foreign, they fight it. Now there's one particular type of cell that's called the helper lymphocyte. The helper lymphocyte seems to be at a crossroads of an awful lot of things that are happening and it is responsible for seeing that the antibodies are good enough, that any cancer cells that might just be generating are fought off, that certain types of rare infections are fought off and that's why you and I don't get thrush. And we don't get these weird things that people who don't have those type of cells have. Now it just so happens that this virus likes those cells. It is a "T" lymphotropic virus. It focuses right on those helper cells and depletes them. Now we know from the natural history of these things that not every cell is going to succumb to them and that cells like this actually can replicate. We're going to find out that there will be people whose "T" cells survive and multiply and recover and that not everyone who has AIDS is going to invariably die from it. That's the good side of the story. And the other good side of the story is that this has been one of the best funded fights against disease ever. The lag time between the discovery of AIDS in 1978 and between the discovery of the virus, and appropriate measures, has been incredibly short. The government has done a marvelous job in following through and taking the lead. If you look at the history of medicine, and you look at the lag times, for instance, in the polio virus, it's infinitely longer. And I think that the anger that often is aroused when something terrible happens, like polio, has to be taken for what it's a sign of: anxiety, or confrontation with the unknown. I think what we're going to have with AIDS, eventually, is a much better understanding of what it is, and the best model for that is the hepatitis B situation in which we just simply know it has to be a direct blood-to-blood contact, or sexual contact with exchanges into the blood of another person by repeated sexual contact. So I hope I've answered some of those questions. . . .

We know that in the United States, in selected areas, there have been more than 12,000 people with AIDS so far. [This was in 1985.] Now think of all the people that these other individuals have come into contact with—thousands of them. They're going to the supermarket, they're going to restaurants, they're going everywhere. Now if it were that contagious, wouldn't we find an epidemic of major proportions which would devastate those cities? No, we haven't seen that. And if you trace those, and the CDC has done just that, the government has traced these individuals, we know how it's transmitted. And there are only the ways that Dr. Grady has been mentioning that represent the true transmission. We know these facts.

Mr. Devine: Dr. Smith, there was a second part to that question. And the second part of the question was, who will monitor the health of the youngster?

Dr. Smith: I will monitor him.

Speaker: Can you tell us about the health of the youngster in the coming year? How you see it progressing?

Dr. Smith: That part of the question is difficult because I have no way of predicting what's going to happen. The worst scenario of AIDS is that there will be one unusual infection after another. These are opportunistic infections and these can take the life of a person. It's an amazing thing about AIDS that AIDS itself does not usually kill, it's the complications of AIDS that kill, like pneumonia, and these other weird things. So I think it's going to have an awful lot to do with identifying these things early enough, so you can treat the complications, and can fend off these infections. And I will be taking care of that, I will be bearing responsibility, along with his other physicians. There are some very fine physicians in the Fall River community who have been doing wonderful work with him. I've been basically managing very closely his hemophilia, but I'm going to also be monitoring him very closely for the other problems as well. So we have a lot of people who are out there working hard for this boy.

Mr. Devine: Other questions? Let me look way up back. Yes, ma'am, right against the wall.

Speaker: My name is Penny B———. I have a daughter at the junior high school. My question is directed to Mr. McCarthy and Mr. Devine. Considering and knowing that the transmission of the disease is through blood and body fluids, hospitals in Fall River and everywhere are utilizing certain procedures for dealing with contact with blood. And if this is policy as it is now, that students or future students who have AIDS are in the school, I don't really understand what you are doing at the junior high school. For instance, let me give you a hypothetical situation, which may seem extreme, but maybe illustrates the case. Suppose a student with AIDS receives a very bad injury of some kind and bleeds, and that student would perhaps fall in the corridor and require assistance. And his friend, who may not know, or another passing student who may not know that this student is carrying the virus, the immediate reaction would be to help the person who's hurt. And in that act of kindness, get blood upon themselves. And if people are anything like me, I always have small cuts on my hands and I've got several now from various things I have done. So within the school environment, knowing that people in hospital situations have to wear gloves and do other certain kinds of procedures, what are you going to do in the junior high school to address those kinds of, perhaps, extreme issues, but they may happen?

Mr. Devine: Mr. McCarthy.

Mr. McCarthy: Well, first of all Penny, just to assure you that in addition to the guidelines that we discussed with regard to attendance in school, also in the guidelines there are directions for school health personnel and that would be our nurse. However, I think the question needs to be answered by a doctor . . . so I'd like to refer that to, perhaps, Dr. Grady?

Dr. Grady: The main thrust of the question first of all has to be: Is there comparability between the hospital setting and the school setting? In other words, why do hospitals have any policies for wearing gloves or gowns at all if there is zero risk? Or, how does that translate into the school? There are several differences. First of all, AIDS is not a disease in the normal sense, as you've heard, it is a weakening of the immune system and the infections that people get superimposed on that system are what lead to a series of events. They may be frequent infections, they may be back to back, there may be a single bout. And it's possible that for this child, as Dr. Smith said, this may be the only infection for a year, or he may have two in a row. That is unpredictable in a given case. But those infections that he gets are with germs that are in this auditorium now and are not new germs to us, and that's not the infection you're worried about.

Now with regard to the hospital setting, the reason the patient is in the hospital is because they are sick, not well. They should not be going to school if they're sick—an obvious difference. The second thing is when they're in the hospital they should require certain procedures, such as drawing blood, doing biopsies, things of that sort, and that's where these gloves and other precautions come in. And they have always existed for other diseases, such as hepatitis, before that. So that is a big difference.

Now I would submit further that there is a possibility, I suppose, for some impulsive act of kindness. But in the situation that we're discussing here now, the child knows that he has an illness, a disability, if you will, that needs careful management, and I assume that he would take some personal responsibility for monitoring his own health if he's bleeding or things of that sort, and that these would be very rare. And in a worse case, as you said, it would require not just dripping of blood on the body or minor cuts. That is probably not a sufficient basis for transmission of this disease as has been demonstrated by the fact that even among medical personnel, even sustaining direct needle sticks, 1000 such people are under follow-up by the CDC right now, and people are looking for these rare instances of transmission. In short, it just isn't that easy to do. So it's a fair question, but I don't think the hospital precautions are transferable as a logical base for anxiety in the school situation under the normal circumstances that we are describing.

Mr. Devine: Procedures, Mrs. B———, procedures which directly address the concern that you raise, are outlined in the policy statements that are available and will be distributed to you before you leave tonight. And those are the ones that are in effect. Sir?

Speaker: My name is Steve B_____ and I have a daughter in the eighth grade and a son in the seventh grade. I'm sure that everybody in this room shares deep compassion for not only the student, but the family. But I for one have become very upset and a little nervous when I hear experts in the medical profession refer to probabilities, when I hear them refer to possibilities that may occur, that may not occur. I think we're losing sight of the fact that we're not dealing with measles, we're not dealing with mumps, we're dealing with a deadly, incurable disease. And what I'd like to know is at what point, or what percentage probability, do you consider acceptable?

Mr. Devine: Thank you. Dr. Smith?

Dr. Smith: I'd like to take that one on. It's a very good question and I think that one of the things that's not taught enough in classrooms is the whole concept of probabilities. . . . I think that a probability is acceptable when it is so infinitesimally small that it probably does not present any significant risk at all of catching something. For instance, I think that the probability of someone after this discussion getting in their car and having a fatal accident is greater than the probability of this child transmitting the disease. That, I think, is how solid the facts are. And those are the types of probabilities that we're talking about in biology. It is extremely remote. . . .

Mr. Devine: Dr. Grady, do you want to respond to that?

Dr. Grady: Yes, I have to go back and say that the range of risks varies from zero to significant in certain circumstances. A sexually active person, in certain settings as we know, has a high risk of AIDS under the circumstances that you have read about. A child sitting next to a child in school under the exact circumstances that have been described here is so close to zero in risk that I can't tell it from zero, if you understand what I'm trying to say. I'm not trying to play God or write insurance policies for anyone. But the only word that comes to mind is "zero" under the settings that we're talking about. That's what I really believe.

Now the minute you start altering the circumstances in saying what if for some reason this child changes his entire behavior pattern? He suddenly shows up in school with a large

ulcer. Other children suddenly start showing up with big open-
ings in their skin, they suddenly get together. You can build a
case where you can make the risks go from zero to something.
But I have to believe that that is nonsense, that that's not what
we're describing here tonight. So under the situation that I
visualize as actually happening in this school, I cannot tell the
risk from zero, that's why I'm using the word.

Speaker: My name is S———— and I have a daughter in the
sixth grade. Doctor, we all know and we all agree that AIDS is
a deadly disease, there is no cure for it. We also agree that it
can be spread to other people through body fluids or other contact. Now can you guarantee me that my daughter, she will not
catch AIDS? I want that 100% guaranteed in writing if you do
so. (*moans from the audience*)

Mr. Devine: Thank you, Mr. S————.

Speaker: I'm not through yet, I want an answer.

Mr. Devine: Is anybody going to give a 100% guarantee in
writing? Do you have another question, Mr. S————?

Speaker: It seems like we're talking in circles here. But we're
talking about a life. And I know what it is because I lost two
childs, I know what it means, so no more laughing please. I
want an answer from the doctor. Can you say that they will not
catch AIDS?

Dr. Smith: Mr. S————, under the circumstances that have
been described here, of a child attending class, sitting next to
another child attending class, I could say that the possibilities
of that happening are zero. (*applause*)

Speaker: So, in other words, if there is such a possibility, the
school committee and the school, doctors as well, are actually
saying to me, Mr. S————, send your daughter to school because if she dies, it's OK, we're proud, we had the first kid in
school. Meanwhile, I go to the girl's funeral. Are you going to
take any responsibility for that?

Mr. Devine: Mr. S————, you asked the doctor if he would
guarantee and the doctor said the possibility is zero. I don't
know what more he can say to you.

Speaker: Well, how come all the doctors in the country, they
disagree with each other? But every one of them says that there
is a possibility to be spread to other people through body fluids

and other contact. How come this will not happen for sure over here at the Case Junior High?

Mr. Devine: Thank you, Mr. S———. Dr. Grady.

Dr. Grady: May I respond? I'm really sorry in a way that the term body fluid gets used because it has one meaning in medicine and another meaning in general use. And I don't blame you for being confused because if one says body fluids, why not assume that sweat and these other things are included? But that's not the intent. I'm telling you that it is bloody fluids, blood-derived serum, that is a means of transmission and there is no evidence otherwise. Now I would not want to insult the gentleman, but I would have to say, can you guarantee me 100% that your daughter would never shoot drugs with another person, or would never have sex with another person? If you can guarantee me that, I can guarantee no AIDS. *(applause)*

Mr. Devine: Thank you, Mr. S———. Are there any further questions? *(Many people start to leave. Some people have been leaving after every speaker.)* I see a hand right near the back of the auditorium. A lady in a white dress.

Speaker: My name is Dee K———. I realize that according to CDC, there are three fluids—blood, serum, especially semen, and saliva—that the AIDS virus has been definitely isolated in. Now if a person has AIDS and goes to the hospital there are some precautions taken. One involves their food trays; everything is disposable, burnt, not recycled. . . . Now you say that probably no one will catch it from saliva or from sputum or whatever. Are our children protected in any way against this? I mean now, does this child eat in the cafeteria using all the school supplies, or does he have to brown bag it? Or are his utensils isolated? Because you can wash these dishes till the cows come home and you're not going to get rid of the virus. It's going to be there, because you're not going to sterilize to get rid of it, not in the school system. I'm just a little concerned, there are 600-plus children in the school who are using these same servings, and to me, I can't feel comfortable with this idea. And I'd just like to know what are some of the physical safeguards being taken for our children in the school?

I work in a hospital, and I work in the laboratory and I know how I have to get dressed in order to handle any of this. I have to put a gown on, I have to put a rubber disposable apron on on top of that, I have to wear two pairs of gloves, I have to wear a filter breathing mask, I have to wear eye goggles, and something on my head. But I realize that I'm coming in direct contact, I'm touching blood. . . . But I don't know that I really feel safe. I know people aren't getting AIDS from casual contact, but the incubation period is six months to five years. That's a long time. There are people out there that are harboring that don't have it yet. And this hemophiliac was diagnosed only because he was one of the high incidence groups. Our children are not necessarily high incidence groups, and how far down the road would we go before we found out? You're not going to go out and donate a pint of blood. So they're not old enough, so they won't get checked for the virus in that manner. And parents aren't going to drag their children to the doctor to have them screened every six months. It's just a very, very scary situation. And I guess we all need an awful lot more reassurance than what is coming out of this panel this evening. *(applause)*

Mr. Devine: Further questions? Sir. *(noise from the audience about not answering the question)* What kinds of safeguards do we have in the school? Thank you.

Dr. Grady: Again, not to be dramatic, but to try to make the point, I have put up a $100 cash reward out of my pocket for the past 20 years for anyone who can show me a food- or water-born transmission of viruses of this family. That reward has gone unclaimed. No one has ever demonstrated the first instance with thousands and millions of people carrying viruses of the hepatitis and herpes family and so forth, and that's in spite of what I would agree with you might be occasional variations in the technique and water temperature and so forth. Even to my surprise, with that variation there has not been transmission through that method. I would further say to you, though, that a common sense precaution might be if a given child who had AIDS or was infected with the virus had bleeding gums or something of that sort, I would certainly not oppose his use of a separate drinking cup or something of that sort. In other words, we're not poo-pooing or outlawing the usual sanitary common sense precautions. But if the normal dishwashing-cleansing procedures are operating with the normal hot water and cleanliness, we have the best, not just theory, but the best evidence in the world that viruses like this cannot be transmitted through that system. It just hasn't happened and people almost would like to see it happen to write about it. They have been looking for it for years. It has not happened, I have no reason to believe it would happen. And I assume that there are checks of the normal, washing-cleanliness policy in the kitchen that do continue here. And I would have to turn back to the school staff to make statements on exactly what those are, but I have no reason to believe that they differ from the usual one.

Dr. Smith: Just a brief comment on what Dr. Grady stated to clarify the hospital policy at Rhode Island Hospital where I work. People who have AIDS, and there have been some, are put on what we call "blood precautions," which is simply guarding against injuring yourself with any bloody articles. So people don't go in there wearing gowns or masks or anything. I think just historically what we have to realize is that when a new disease is discovered, there is just a tremendous amount of uncertainty as to how it is spread, and the normal common sense guideline is to protect yourself very much, particularly those workers who are coming in direct contact with the agent. And this is particularly the lab workers. My feeling is that probably what we are going to be seeing is a loosening of those criteria. Just as I don't gown or mask or do anything but wash my hands when I deal with a patient, with any patient for that matter, including those with AIDS. I have the feeling that the safe practices which are common sense may very well change in the hospital environment, including the laboratory environment, as more is understood about that. But as long as you are in direct contact with the possible agent, those precautions in the laboratory are generally stricter than in the hospital ward. But remember that the hospital ward in "blood precautions" uses normal dishes.

Mr. Devine: Mr. McCarthy.

Mr. McCarthy: Yes, the hot water is monitored. It is the correct temperature for washing. There is a mandated temperature. I can't tell you exactly what it is, but it is monitored and we do take safeguards to see that everything is washed properly with the proper temperature of water.

Mr. Devine: Sir. *(Many people get up and leave.)*

Speaker: My name is Vic B————. I have a daughter in the seventh grade, I'm from Swansea. This debate can go on all night long; it's like a tennis match. And you gentlemen have a slight advantage because you're all polished because you've gone to school probably twice as long as us. And you have a way with words. Dr. Grady, you keep saying "zero ground" and Dr. Smith has a favorite word "possibilities." I would like just two answers and I'd like them with a simple yes or a simple no. Can you guarantee 100% (*some moans from the audience*) that no one will ever catch AIDS here? That's all I'm asking. And if they do, if one person does, I want a simple answer, yes or no, was it worth it?

Dr. Grady: All right, I'd be glad to go first. First of all I don't know why you want to make fun of my ability to answer your questions. I'm proud of my education and I hope that everyone in this school gets a good one, too. (*loud applause*)

Speaker: But you have a way with words! And you . . .

Dr. Grady: I can also tell the truth, though, with a way with words, and I'm telling you the truth and resent any indication that I'm not.

Speaker: And I resent, too, the fact that you're using big words and this is a simple thing, make it plain and simple, yes or no!

Dr. Grady: I've already stated, I will state again, if your child, and again no offense to you, I hope should never have sexual contact or share needles with a child with AIDS. . . . (*He is interrupted.*)

Speaker: We're not talking needles or sex, we're talking 100% guarantee that no one's child will get AIDS! Not zero ground, 100%!

Dr. Grady: No, you're . . . (*interrupted again*)

Speaker: That's what I'm talking, don't give me "no use" because you can't get out of it! I want an answer!

Dr. Grady: I'm giving you . . . (*interrupted again*)

Speaker: You can't give me one!

Dr. Grady: I'm giving you one . . . (*interrupted again*)

Speaker: You can't give me one because they don't have one yet!

Mr. Devine: Why don't you let Dr. Grady try to answer your question? You've asked it 17 times and he can't answer it yet!

Speaker: He's gonna double talk me! He's gonna double talk me! Yes or no? I went to high school, but I understand yes or no. I'm not polished, but I know what yes means.

Mr. Devine: Thank you. Dr. Grady.

Dr. Grady: I will repeat my answer. I see no risk, I see zero risk in the absence of conditions which *you* have to guarantee and I don't see why you want to escape that responsibility? (*applause*)

Mr. Devine: Are there any further questions? Sir.

Last Speaker: Where's my answer? Can you guarantee nobody will get it? (*moans from the audience*)

Dr. Grady: No child will contract AIDS in the absence of the exceptional types of contact which each parent must bear the responsibility for. Sitting next to the child, no. Playing with the child, no. 100% No! No! No! (*loud applause*)

Last Speaker: We're not talking sitting next to, we're talking something that is unforeseen. You don't know, I don't like to take things from the newspapers or the movie actresses who refuse to kiss movie actors now because they say deep kissing can bring it on. (*moans from the audience*) That's what they're saying. So what's the difference between deep kissing and a sneeze? It's still saliva. (*talking going on in the audience*)

Mr. Devine: Thank you. Sir.

Speaker: My name is Robert C———. (*talking still going on in the audience*) I live in Swansea.

Mr. Devine: Excuse me, Mr. C———, could you hold on a minute please? I'm sure people can't hear you.

Speaker: I have a boy in the seventh grade. I've been listening to what I guess you could say is a good public forum and I appreciate you folks coming down here to help us out. I want to address a couple of things that have come up here tonight. Number one, Dr. Smith has said that AIDS is not an epidemic. OK. This is the *Providence Journal*, September 1: "In New York City where AIDS has outdistanced murder, suicide, and cancer as the number one killer of men age 30–39, hospital workers have been accused of shunning AIDS patients, for fear of contracting the disease." I have one more, *Providence Journal*: "Is AIDS fatal? Eventually yes, half of its victims are now dead. Is AIDS spreading? Yes, the number of cases is expected to double

this year." Item number B which we talked about tonight. I'd
like to quote Dr. Grady who said, "The rights of the majority
should not be subordinated to the rights of the minority."

Dr. Grady: That's correct.

Speaker: OK, so let's look at the report which you held up
to everyone. (*He shows the crowd.*) I've read this report, it just
came in the mail today from the CDC, Center for Disease Control. Again, I'm addressing the Item B which you recommended
that we not inform children, not hold an auditorium meeting
and inform the children. From this report which Dr. Grady
held up, the title of it is from the Center for Disease Control,
August 30, 1985, and it's entitled: "Morbidity and Mortality,
Weekly Report, Section 517, Education and Foster Care of Children Infected with the AIDS Virus. . . . All educational and
public health departments," this is paragraph 11, "All educational and public health departments, regardless of whether
the AIDS infected children are involved, are strongly encouraged
to inform parents, children, and educators involving the AIDS
virus and its transmission. Such education would greatly as-
sist efforts to provide the best care and education for infected
children while minimizing the risk of transmission to others."

I'd like to read one more on this issue. From the *Providence
Journal* again, Dr. Kenneth H. Maher, an infectious disease specialist—AIDS is an infectious disease—at Memorial Hospital,
Pawtucket, and part of the AIDS Advisory Committee to the
Health Department, believes "schools should immediately begin programs to educate children to the dangers of AIDS, particularly adolescents on the verge of becoming sexually active." This is where I feel we should inform the children. This
is not my opinion, my opinion doesn't matter, but these are
opinions of learned men such as yourself.

Item C, Transmission Possibilities. Again quoting this report that you waved to the people, but didn't read. Paragraph
4: "Care involving exposure to the infected Child's Body Fluids
and Excrement." By the way, one of the symptoms that you
know you have AIDS is diarrhea, that's in the article there, diarrhea and swelling and different things. OK. "Care involving the
exposure to the infected child's body fluids and excrements
should be performed by persons who are aware of the child's
infection and modes of possible transmission." Paragraph 5: "be-

cause other infections in addition to AIDS can be present in blood or body fluids, all schools, regardless of whether children with AIDS infection are attending, should adapt routine procedures for handling blood and body fluids." I want to know what our children know about this? Should there be a blood spill near them, are they going to grab a paper towel and help the teacher clean it up? What do the janitors know about this? OK. It says, "those who are cleaning should avoid exposure of their own open skin lesions or mucous membranes." So if you're cleaning this up, you shouldn't touch your nose, because that's an open area of your body. OK.

My last item on the transmission of the AIDS virus. This is from the same report, volume 34, which states, now what I'm really trying to get at here is that number one, we should inform our children and parents of AIDS, of the ways you can contract it, with a forum, with a meeting for the children. OK. That's number one. Number two, I really believe there should be precautions spelled out, not just to the teachers, but to the children, like "stay away from this." If this happens, the child is a bleeder, so it won't be a little bit of blood, it might be a lot of blood, if he should get cut in gym, or something like that. OK.

Now I feel an ounce of precaution is worth a pound of cure. I didn't invent that. But these are recommendations from the CDC, for preventing possible transmission of the AIDS virus from tears. Now this just came out this month, August 30. OK? This is really addressed to the medical profession because they're also, we've talked to many doctors who are concerned about the spread of this virus and they feel that if we're going to err, we should err on the side of safety. OK? OK, now this item written by the CDC addressing medical type people said, "the etiological agent of AIDS has been found in various body fluids, including blood, semen, saliva. Recently scientists at the National Institute of Health isolated the virus in tears. The following precautions," and that's all I ask for, precautions, here, "the following precautions are judged suitable to prevent the spread of the AIDS virus that might be present in tears," and I might add other body fluids, "precautions: 1) health care professionals performing eye examinations involving contact with tears should wash their hands immediately after procedure

and between patients. Hand washing alone should be sufficient, but where practical and convenient, disposable gloves
may be worn. And the use of gloves is advisable especially
where there are cuts, or scratches, or lesions on the hands of
the person who is caring for the AIDS person."

So the point I'm trying to make here is that I don't feel, I
don't feel right now enough is being done. I think these learned
people here have made a good point. This has all come out in
the past two weeks. These studies saying, look, it's going to
double in a year. More people are dying from it in New York
City, between the ages of 30 and 39, than from cancer and murder, and other diseases put together. OK. So it is an epidemic,
Dr. Smith, as far as I'm concerned, in my eyes it's an epidemic,
OK? So why don't we practice excessive cautions in this case,
establish procedures, tell the children the dangers, tell them
the precautions, let's inform everyone. And I feel that if we do
that, we'll go a long way toward alleviating a lot of people's
fears. People want to worry about paper plates and things like
that. You mentioned that that's maybe not necessary, right?
But it doesn't cost much to give the child some paper plates
and forks and it makes people feel at ease. And you're not worried about handling these types of things and washing them.
OK? Even the people in the food handlers' department in the
kitchen it kind of puts them at ease and doesn't cost much. So
these are the kinds of things that I think, I feel are important.
Thank you very much for the floor. *(applause)*

Mr. Devine: Thank you, Mr. C———. Dr. Smith.

Dr. Smith: All of us here have taken this case very seriously.
We have taken special measures to try to inform the people
who would be in the management and daily care of this child.
The business about the transmission from the tears, I think,
is more or less a situation which we've talked about. It's one
thing having the virus and it's another thing talking about the
transmission of the virus. And I agree that safe precautions
should be taken and they are being taken in the hospital environment. And I think that the guidelines as outlined here in
the CDC communication are very relevant in that regard.

In terms of the confidentiality issue, I just wanted to draw
your attention to page 518, in which they do mention how important it is to preserve the confidentiality and privacy in this

particular setting. Because with AIDS goes a lot of labeling, as you can well imagine. And everybody, if they're not going to do harm, has a right to their own privacy. And I think this explains why we took the approach that we did take. We started with a small group, and because of all these happenings, these things snowballing with the New York School District and the Indiana events, and things like that, we felt that it was more or less inevitable that we'd have to speak to larger and larger groups. But in doing so, I personally fear that we may be drawing so much attention to this issue, that it may, in the long run, violate privacy and confidentiality. And remember, read that section again about confidentiality because it is very important.

And the other thing about education of children—I think that's a very relevant point. When I came to speak with the teachers the other day, I mentioned if you ever wanted to bring it up, do so by asking how does the normal body defend against invaders. Now that would be a very interesting subject because the whole business about what AIDS is is buried in that whole thing. But try to give a good overview of immunity, and then discuss it from there. Thank you.

Mr. Devine: Further questions? From someone we haven't heard from yet. Yes, ma'am.

Speaker: Thank you, Mr. Devine, my hand was getting tired. My name is Jean S———. I'm from Swansea and I have six children and four grandchildren. And, yes, I am very afraid of this disease that I don't understand. And from what I've heard, I don't really think anybody does understand. But first of all, what I want to say is as far as compassion, I'm not here because of the boy, I'm here because of the disease. It has nothing to do with the family or anything else, and I don't want to be in their place in six months or five years, and that's why I'm here. My question is for Dr. Smith. Are we really doing him a favor by letting him in school? If the immunity system is attacked and he has no immunity, somebody who sneezes next to him, it could be fatal to him, where for the boy or the girl, it could be just a cold. But to him, it could be fatal. Are we doing him a favor?

Mr. Devine: Thank you, Mrs. S———. Dr. Smith.

Dr. Smith: Yes, we are, simply because the type of infections these children get are so very specific and they're so very rare that they're not from common colds and sneezes. Actually, in fact, I don't know of any cases, maybe Dr. Grady knows of some, in which they've even caught disseminated chicken pox, or things like that. It seems to be very specific types of infections caused by fungi, or by organisms that are called protozoa, that they're particularly prone to. Particularly in the hemophilia population—and that's one of the mysteries that we don't really understand—why this specificity? Why is it just these particular organisms? So I don't worry about his welfare in the school system. And, believe me, I would be the first one to keep him out of school if I thought it would do him harm.

Mr. Devine: Further questions? Yes, sir. Yes, Mr. M———.

Speaker: You can hear my voice?

Mr. Devine: Mr. M———, please wait for a mike so that the TV can pick you up.

Speaker: You know it's a shame that we live in a world where we need guarantees. But I'll ask for a guarantee. If this boy was removed from the school system, OK, would you be able to give a guarantee that my daughter still would not come down with AIDS? *(applause)* Thank you.

Mr. Devine: Further questions? Yes, ma'am.

Speaker: My name is Kathleen L———. I have a son in the seventh grade. He works in the cafeteria, in fact, he handles all the trays. I feel that all my questions have been answered. I thank you and I feel safe letting him go to school. *(applause)*

Mr. Devine: Thank you, Mrs. L———. Let me try to call on people who haven't been heard from yet. Sir, on the aisle, white shirt.

Speaker: Hi, my name is Dan G———. And I'd just like to say personally my prayers go out to the family of that young man and I share the feelings that you must have for your situation. Obviously, you gentlemen on the panel and the State Board of Education and Public Health are breaking some new ground here. We're going to be in a fish bowl in this community for many years, as long as the young man is in school. This is not a situation that is going to go away overnight. I'm one of those parents that is looking for some sort of reassurance. Something that would probably help is to ask the question, do you have any plans to monitor all the children in the school medically as this child progresses through school?

Dr. Grady: Well, I think that the decision about what normal monitoring should be is something that should be decided by the school health physicians. But all I can say is that the Department of Public Health will make available any and every technical type of assistance. If, after consideration, people feel that there is evidence that an unusual number of children are sick, or something funny is going on, obviously, we will investigate it. We do that every day, regardless of whether it's known or unknown, or suspected that disease X or Y is there.

I'm in charge of the state laboratories as well as the investigations, and we'll make every type of support available that makes sense. But I don't think we should start a witch hunt right away and start suggesting to people, gee, don't you feel a little funny? I mean, after all, your parents came to a meeting tonight and we talked about AIDS. I mean, I think that will really backfire and so I think we have to be careful about suggesting it. And there have been several well-documented cases, or epidemics if you will, of hysterical disease. I know it sounds silly, but it's especially prevalent in junior high schools. Junior high students are of an age when they are especially susceptible to suggestions. And there have been waves of people passing out or vomiting or whatever, purely based on that sort of thing. So that's part of what worries me and I think that the children will pick up from their parents a level of expectation as to whether this is normal or risky. And that's why I feel privileged to come here tonight, and do my best to tell you how we feel and why we feel it. And that it's my personal belief that this is a situation that is completely manageable on the basis of good information.

Speaker: OK, thank you. One other question on that. I understand that we would be the first school system that would allow a child with AIDS. Is that correct?

Dr. Grady: No, that's not correct.

Speaker: OK, thank you.

Dr. Grady: Actually New York has had a child in school for more than three years, but they did not discuss it with the people that were involved. And my suspicion is, based on national statistics, that there are a good number of children with AIDS in schools. I feel that what's unique here is that there was a genuine attempt to deal with this up front, head on, short of identifying the child, which was synonymous with a media parade . . . with a proper sequence of discussion with teachers and those who need to know why a child may need to be out or in school. So I think that's what's unique, that this has been a cooperative effort with school and health people. But no, I don't think that this is the only child in the United States in school with AIDS.

Speaker: Thank you very much, I appreciate it.

Mr. Devine: Thank you, Mr. G———. Yes, ma'am, I see a green sleeve. Yes, ma'am.

Speaker: My name is Doris M——— and my son just entered the junior high this year. I have sort of a two-fold question. The first part is, why are we the scapegoats for the whole country? Our little corner of the world seems to be the one that everyone is focusing on. We're the ones who are going to allow this to happen. Then what's going to happen? Everyone's going to turn their back. The illustrious medical review board has malpractice insurance. We can't go against them if something happens. Second question, I have basically, not total information, but some information that I've gotten, it states that AIDS is a virus, that it is not necessarily rampant, but yet it doesn't show up for another two to five years. So what's going to happen in the two years between that time when our children then come down with the susceptibilities necessary to put them in the same situation that this child is in now? I'd still like to know what's happening to our tax dollar that we're paying these educators to evaluate what's going to happen with us and then tell us after the horse is out of the barn?

Mr. Devine: Mr. McCarthy, do you want to respond to any of that?

Mr. McCarthy: Well, first of all, I think Dr. Grady made some mention of the fact about the number of children in the country who have AIDS. There was a little different approach that we took. This educator that you are paying, you're paying him to make hard decisions based on advice and facts that come from experts. The decision that was made relied on the public health people to define whether he should or should not go to school. That was not my decision, it was a public health decision. And somebody has to make those decisions. And secondly, my role in this was to follow the law and provide the rights for the individual student. And I'd like to do the same for your child, if he or she was unfortunate enough to be in either this kind of a situation, or some other situation. That's the responsibility of this educator that your taxes are paying for. (*applause*)

Mr. Devine: Further questions? Yes, ma'am.

Speaker: My name is Carol G———. Apparently, since it was already decided that the boy will stay in school, that decision was made before we got here, so I guess we're going to have to live with it. I'd like to think that what we're doing is minimizing the risks as much as possible. I'd like to know, and I'd like the answer from you please, Mr. Devine, because it's your school that the boy is in and our children are in, I'd like to know what precautions are being taken to minimize the risks as much as possible. Keeping in mind, that it is in tear ducts, it is in saliva, it is in body fluids. Keeping in mind that the boy is 13 years old and we know how 13-year-old boys can be. You know, is he taking care of himself? Is he well aware of the situation? Does he know the proper way to behave? For example, the superintendent in Indiana, they decided in Indiana that they wouldn't let the boy in and the superintendent said, what are we going to do about someone chewing pencils, sneezing, and swimming in the pool? Fortunately, we don't have a pool, but you know, there is the sneezing and swimming. Is the boy well aware of the situation to be able to handle his own hygiene habits and so on that he can monitor himself? Is there somebody else involved participating that can watch over him? I don't even know if at the junior high school we use paper plates, or what we use, but, you know, if we don't use paper plates, is somebody trying to insure and minimize the damage? And the second part of that is where there are the possibilities like he really shouldn't be coming when he has a severe cold . . . open sores . . . so on. . . . Is the nurse involved, or who's involved? I'd really like you to answer these questions.

Mr. Devine: I'll answer them. I'll answer them.

Speaker: I know at the hospitals they have precautions.

Mr. Devine: OK, to answer question number one, we are dealing with a very responsible youngster. The youngster is bright and he's articulate, he's very knowledgeable about his condition. And he is quite capable of monitoring his conditions and sending out the danger signs, so to speak, if any condition were to exist that would be cause for concern. So, we're dealing with a highly responsible eighth grade youngster.

Number two, who will monitor him if he becomes ill? I believe you asked who would be determining just when he would continue to come to school or who would make the decision as to whether he should be excluded from school—that would be his attending physician, one of whom is Dr. Smith. The state regulations dictate that that decision is a medical one. And Dr. Smith, I think, just from our experience here tonight and my several contacts with him, certainly has all my confidence. He would never place his patient in a position of jeopardy. He would never place our children in a position of jeopardy, either. So the medical decision will be made by the medical people. The responsibility that we would have a right to expect from a youngster so afflicted has been shown by this youngster and he is a very responsible youngster.

You alluded to cafeteria utensils. The utensils that are used in the cafeteria are all disposable. We do not re-use any utensils. They do eat off trays and the trays are cleaned. Mr. McCarthy mentioned some time ago that the actual cleaning process is governed by regulations and our cleaning process meets those regulations. I don't know what more I can say. Yes, ma'am, right behind.

Speaker: Hello, my name is Beverly M———— and I have a child that attends Case Junior High School. First of all, we hear Mr. McCarthy saying constantly, the rights of this child, fine, nobody's disagreeing that this child should have an education, but what about the rights of our children? We have a panel up there who say in their opinion it's not dangerous, our children can't catch it. My own physician says, no way, to let that child go to school. So, it's just a matter of opinion. Why not take another alternative? Why not keep this child home and give him the education at home and not take this risk of putting our children through all this? How do any of these panel know that our children haven't already got it? How do you know that? How do we know it? We don't know it. Like we said, there's 12,000 people in the United States confirmed. But what about the ones who are not confirmed? What about the ones who have it and they don't know they have it? Why should we jeopardize the lives of our children for one child? I sympathize with them. I come from a family of 17 children. I have all the sympathy in the world for this child, but not more than for my own child. (*applause*)

Mr. Devine: Thank you, Mrs. M———. Mr. McCarthy, would you like to respond to that?

Mr. McCarthy: Yes, I'll respond to the first part of the question where we're talking about the rights of the individual or the rights of the many. In the first place, unless there is a determined risk, and that's determined by the public health people, then the right of the individual states that that child has a right to go to school. There has not been any verified public risk. I'm going by regulation, law, and the people in public health who are supposed to make that decision. There is no risk. This is what the regulation says. Therefore, the right of the individual has to be protected.

Speaker: But haven't they been wrong a number of times? And they can be wrong again a number of times. This is a new disease. There isn't enough known about it!

Mr. Devine: Excuse me, Mrs. M———. I believe that Mr. McCarthy did respond to your concern. We'll be happy to come back to you later. Sir?

Speaker: Hi. My name is Reggie Desnoyers [Mark's Little League manager]. I feel especially interested in this thing, because the boy in question played for me in Little League for three years. In due respect to my friend Lenny C——— in the back, he's partially wrong. This boy played for me when he was 10, 11, and this year until he became ill sometime in June. It wasn't until about the first of July that I became aware of the disease that he really had. I had quite a conversation with the father about it, who happened to be one of my coaches. And he gave me all the information that Dr. Smith has given us here. Without ever meeting Dr. Smith prior to tonight, knowing the father, knowing the family, knowing how high class they are, how trustworthy they are, I accepted it the way it was. July the 4th, I snuck into the hospital, through a back door, to visit the boy and I'm proud of it! The boy was in my daughter's class last year, I have a daughter 12 years old, I have seven children of my own. I am very close to that family. As a matter of fact I spent three hours there Sunday night. I spent two hours there Thursday night. I love my daughter, I'm not worried about her catching a disease. Now aren't people here barking up the wrong limb, Doc? Isn't this disease more communicable through sex and drug addiction through hypodermic needles? How many people here allow their children out till 2 or 3 o'clock in the morning? Probably half-bombed with alcohol, the real social problem in our day and age — drugs! (*applause*) And then what goes on? That's the way they can catch AIDS, not by playing hide-and-go-seek with a kid, that believe me, I'm proud to know. (*applause*)

Mr. Devine: Further comments? Again, I'd like to go to someone we haven't heard from yet. Yes, ma'am.

Speaker: Hello, my name is Shirley R———. I heard the boy has a sister who also has the blood disease, is that true?

Mr. Devine: That's not true. Further questions? Yes, ma'am.

Speaker: My name is Rosetta P——— and I have a daughter in this school. My question is to all of you sitting out there. Mr. McCarthy, do not be upset when you see a scared parent out here like I am asking you a question. I don't know this child who has the disease. My daughter knows him and I've kept my child at home since Friday, since I knew what happened. She says, "Ma, I want to go, I love that kid, he's a nice kid." Yes, I feel very much for him and his parents, but I also have a right to protect my child. And it is a deadly disease, isn't it, Dr. Smith? Dr. Grady, isn't it a deadly disease? Can you tell me really it isn't? I will drop my body in front of a car to protect my child! I am not going to send my child to school. As much as I feel for these parents and this kid, I will not send my daughter to school while I know that there is a deadly disease in the school. I am very sorry, and I do appreciate from the bottom of my heart all of you here trying to tell us and educate us about the disease. But none of you can guarantee us. There is many parents who are out here, I know they all feel the way I do. I am shaking because I have never taken a mike this big, and I'd never do that, but when it comes to my child, I will speak in front of anybody and tell you that I will not send my child to school — not until this is all cleared. Thank you.

Mr. Devine: Thank you, Mrs. P———. Is there any further discussion?

Speaker: I'm Terry P——— from Swansea and I'd like to direct my question to either doctor who can answer it. I'd like to know if all the people who are carrying the AIDS virus, are they all in the high risk group?

Dr. Grady: I'm sorry, could you repeat the question?

Speaker: I asked if all the people that are carrying the AIDS antibodies, are they all in the high risk groups?

Dr. Grady: Well, first of all, the antibodies mean that that person has encountered the virus at some earlier point in time. And only a fraction of those who have antibody are in fact still carrying the virus, some have thrown it off. So, it's hard for me to answer the question as you asked it, because the first half is not quite right. In other words, the antibody per se is not a measure of being a carrier, regardless of what group you are in. Now of those who have antibodies, they are concentrated in the high risk groups—the second part of your question.

Speaker: So where did the carriers get the antibodies?

Dr. Grady: The theory as to the origin of AIDS is the same as the theory for the other diseases of western civilization, whether it be smallpox, or hepatitis, or whatever. These viruses arise and mutate in nature, either through animal systems, monkeys, chimpanzees in the jungles, whatever. They gradually evolve through a process of evolutions and adapt to new animal systems that can support their growth, because they cannot exist independently in nature. So the theory, for all of these diseases, and sometimes they can be tracked backwards actually to their origin, is that they evolve either from animal populations to humans or from human populations that are in sequestered parts of the world. The best theory for the source of AIDS is that it arose in Central Africa and somehow found its way through the Caribbean into the United States.

Speaker: I'm aware of where it arose from, what I'm asking you is that the people who have AIDS antibodies in their blood, didn't they get them from someone else who had AIDS?

Dr. Grady: They got them from someone else who was carrying the virus, but they may or may not have had AIDS. That's the only reason I'm hesitating to answer your question, the way you asked it.

Speaker: Somehow I feel you're being evasive. (*She laughs.*)

Dr. Grady: I'm doing the best I can, but I can't answer an incorrect question; that would make the answer incorrect. I'm sorry.

Speaker: Well, how do you explain the incidents of the AIDS carriers in Zaire and Florida? They have found carriers that are not in the high risk groups.

Dr. Grady: As I tried to explain there are parts of the world where the virus may develop early on, transmitted from mother to child, for example, and may be present, in a modified form that may be very mild so that it doesn't surface until it gets into other types of populations that have never seen it before, then it becomes expressed. There probably always was hepatitis B in Asia and Africa for centuries, but only in this century, in the 1900s, has it been recognized in the United States. Probably because of the transfer of one population that handles it differently into another population that expresses it. Am I making sense now?

Speaker: No. (*laughter*)

Dr. Grady: Sorry.

Speaker: You mentioned that families were tested and none of the family members have contracted AIDS. What about the incubation period which I heard was anywhere from six months to 10 years? Not many children have been involved and for so little time. Can you really base this conclusion of it not being spread casually from such a short period of time that it's been actually researched?

Dr. Grady: First of all, the range that you mention is a little extreme. In children, the only accurate estimates of so-called incubation periods would come from when you knew that the mother is the source and the child contracted it at birth.

Speaker: Well, I'm talking about hemophiliac children that are living at home.

Dr. Grady: OK, but in general, the incubation period would be perhaps six months, a year or so. So there have been opportunities for several generations of transmission to have taken place, if they were going to, if that's the question you're asking.

Speaker: Well, I've heard the incubation period to be six months to 10 years.

Dr. Grady: No, the 10 years is incorrect. The longest ever seen was: A) not in children B) following transfusions. And that is in extreme, out to four or five years, but I don't know of any 10 years.

Speaker: Thank you.

Mr. Devine: Any further questions? Yes, ma'am.

Speaker: My name is Debra T———— and I'd like to know what's being done now to find a cure for AIDS, and how close we are to finding a cure?

Dr. Grady: Well, I think Dr. Smith and I would both like to answer that. And, in fact, I would suggest to him maybe a better analogy, since he deals with not only hemophilia and blood diseases, but certain cancers and cancers of the bloodstream, including leukemia and lymphomas. It wasn't that long ago, perhaps a decade ago, when if a child contracted leukemia, it was a source of great sadness because very few children recovered or survived. Now, as I understand, there are certain forms of childhood leukemia that approximately 50% are getting, I don't want to call it a cure, but a permanent remission. In other words, they return to health. And all that over the course of a decade. Now during that process, children who had far advanced disease probably were not as hopeful of having a benefit from any of the new treatments that were then under study. Now there are at least 10 different types of drugs being looked at for AIDS. And I would say that a child who is near death's door has very little chance of benefiting because that research won't be completed. But if you take a child who is just presenting the first manifestation of AIDS, as is the case that we are talking about here, I think there is a fairly good chance that one or more of the treatments now under study may be proven out before that child's case is too advanced. I don't want to put a percentage on it, but it is not a hopeless case by any means.

Mr. Devine: Further questions? Yes, ma'am.

Speaker: I'd like to address this to Dr. Smith.

Mr. Devine: Would you state your name and address, please.

Speaker: Susan B————. I'd like to know what kind of infections this young man might be getting, like within the next maybe six months or so? And will they affect the health of other children in the school?

Dr. Smith: Thank you for the question. The most common type of infection that is seen in people with hemophilia with AIDS is what they call PCP or pneumocystis carinii pneumonia. This is a very rare type of pneumonia that was originally described in pediatric literature in premature infants, so you see how rare it is. Because it's been around for a long time and been described in these prematures, we know for a fact that it is not contagious. You can't catch it from one person to another, so that kind of pneumonia is definitely not contagious. The other types of infections that have occurred in people with hemophilia have been some of the rare type of fungi. And they can get into the central nervous system, for instance, and cause meningitis. But that again is a totally noncommunicable type of disease. And were he to get any one of these conditions, believe me, he wouldn't be here, he wouldn't be able to get out of bed.

Speaker: One other question, what makes a person a carrier of AIDS? I mean, do you have to be a certain type of person? Do you have to have a certain blood type, or how do you carry it?

Dr. Smith: The medical definition of being a carrier is that you have the virus particle in your blood, yet you're not sick from it. Get me?

Speaker: Yes.

Dr. Smith: So probably for all the people who actually have AIDS, there are probably other people who actually carry the germ without any sickness. Unfortunately, because the virus is so incredibly fastidious and difficult to culture, the number of carriers who have actually been detected are in very small numbers. This is very hard to culture and it takes literally weeks and weeks to try to get it. And each time you try to culture the virus, the chance of the batch dying off are very great. And the cost of doing a viral culture for the AIDS virus is about $1,000 a shot. So, what I'm saying is that we don't have enough information to answer that question, but there probably are areas . . .

Dr. Grady: Could I answer it briefly, too? And be as simple as possible. First of all, I like the question because whereas I feel that we know so much about the means of transmission, you just put your finger on the 64 million dollar question. We do not know why some people react to any virus, resolve the infection completely and throw it off. Others get sick, not sick, or some actually come to peace with it and it parasitizes their bodies and lives in a funny type of false harmony with their system. And that is an example of the part that we don't understand, not only about AIDS, but about other virus diseases. And those are the kinds of medical studies for which Nobel

Prizes are being given right now. So it's a very complicated and very important question and the answer is, we don't know.

Speaker: Is that part of the reason why some people carry cancer cells?

Dr. Grady: That's correct. The reason why some people carry cancer cells, in theory, is that there is a scavenger system, a defense system, that is circulating all the time that detects foreign invaders, whether it be cancerous changes or particles from the outside. And sometimes that system goes down and goes out of balance. And studying the reasons for that is the task of the science of immunology—that's a whole field—and that's where most of the breakthroughs are being made today.

Mr. Devine: Further questions? Yes, ma'am.

Speaker: My name is Debra F———. My question is directed to Mr. McCarthy. Since this student is being allowed to enter school now, is it going to be a policy where any child that has AIDS is going to be allowed to enter the Swansea school system?

Mr. McCarthy: The policy that will be followed is the policy that has been established by the Department of Education and also by Public Health. That's the policy and that's what I'm following.

Speaker: What about kindergarten students or first graders? With the younger children I hear that there is a higher risk.

Mr. McCarthy: I'll turn this over to the Department of Education.

Mr. Hall: I agree with Mr. McCarthy's statement that it's the policy of the Commonwealth of Massachusetts of both the Public Health and Education. Each case is an individual case and that's the policy. So the fact that this child is effectively, appropriately, placed in school, should not be construed that each and every child automatically will be placed in school. That a child will be placed in school requires, first, an appropriate medical determination that it's right to be in school, and then we at the Department of Education will in fact expect that whatever school department receives that child will provide for an appropriate educational service. On the other hand, we at the Education Department assume that the medical profession, we not only assume, we know, that they will simply not send to us a child that is not appropriate in school. So the policy is not a blanket policy. It's a policy that says each and every case will be determined on the specifics of that case. So it may well be that some other child may contract this disease and not be admitted to school. . . .

Speaker: Aren't the risks higher with younger children though? Because of the way they handle themselves as far as going to the bathroom and spitting, and that type of thing— biting.

Mr. Devine: Dr. Smith.

Dr. Smith: The statement that was issued under discussion and which you've seen right here actually mentions certain qualifications. And there are two things that are specifically targeted in this statement. For smaller children, in which there is a possibility of not handling their secretions appropriately, or biting or something like that, it is considered prudent and good practice to avoid integration of that child into a school. In terms of the susceptibility of the other children in the kindergarten age group, I don't believe it to be significantly different from any type of child. The types of children who actually get these crazy types of infections are basically premature babies and infants who are at somewhat of a disadvantage. But school age children and kindergarten age children are not at any greater risk.

Mr. Devine: Mrs. F———, the guidelines which you will receive before leaving tonight also directly address the issues that you are raising. Further questions? Sir.

Speaker: My name is Allan A———. I have four school age children, the oldest is in the junior high school. The younger of the children, the other three, go to E.S. Brown. I have sort of a two-part, two-fold question. I understand that the child with the AIDS disease is currently in the hospital and has been in the hospital for several days. Could you elaborate as to his current medical status as it stands and also when he will be returning to school in his current condition? And secondly, I understand also that this child's brother is a fifth grade student at the E.S. Brown School and also has the condition of hemophilia. I would like your medical status on this child, Dr. Smith. Thank you.

Dr. Smith: I will try to answer your question without it violating confidentiality, which is very dear to my heart. First of all, I think it's safe to say that he is not in the hospital since if he were in the hospital, he would be in my care. Currently, if he's out of school, it is because of hemophilia. As I mentioned before, it happens as simply a matter of course that people with hemophilia bleed spontaneously, and generally into their joints and into their muscles, and this can happen anytime and it just happens to be his bad luck.

As to his brother, he's healthy, happy, doing well. In fact, both of the kids have been participating this summer, as you know, in all kinds of activities and the boy in question has been very active in Little League activities, and learning golf, and all those sorts of things. So, apart from the fact that he's suffering from his hemophilia right now, he seems to be doing all right.

Mr. Devine: Further questions? Anyone that I've not heard from? Sir.

Speaker: My name is Steve B———. I have a question for Dr. Grady. Earlier in a response to a question, you referred to a student in the New York school system that had apparently been there for three years. To your knowledge, since he has been there for three years, have any other students in his class contracted AIDS and if so . . .

Dr. Grady: No! No!

Speaker: They haven't. Thank you.

Mr. Devine: Thank you, Mr. B———. Further questions? Sir.

Speaker: I have two questions. First of all . . .

Mr. Devine: Would you state your name and address please.

Speaker: Dave R———. My son attends the seventh grade at the school. The first question I have is, is there anyone here representing the Massachusetts Board of Health? I was just wondering, or if they know what the Massachusetts Board of Health has stated on this issue?

Dr. Grady: Yes, I am the assistant commissioner of the Massachusetts Department of Public Health. The policy which has been handed out is a policy developed by the Department of Public Health, endorsed by the governor's task force, and shared and endorsed by the Department of Education as well. That's what you're supposed to have made available to you, that's it.

Speaker: The second part of my question is to Mr. McCarthy. I'm sure what he's done is he's followed the policy of the state.

He's made his decision in good conscience with the help of educated people in the field that were talking out there. The question that I have is that we know that a similar incident has taken place in Indiana, where probably a very good superintendent made a similar decision, only his decision was not to allow that student to attend. And I'll quote the statement that was made when he decided not to admit that student because "it posed too much of a risk to other students." He points to "warnings from the Indiana Board of Health about the risks of the exposure to AIDS through infected saliva and body fluids." Now who are we to assume is the inferior Board of Health?

Mr. McCarthy: I don't think we need to infer either as an inferior Board of Health. But the Board of Health in the state of Massachusetts has made a different recommendation. As a matter of fact, you're reading a quote and I don't know indeed what that regulation is in the state of Indiana. And I don't know why that superintendent made his decision. I attempted to explain to you why I made a decision here. And I will not, I will not evaluate him, as I hope my colleague will not evaluate me.

Speaker: That's not my point. I don't think you made a wrong decision based on the information you were given. What I am saying is that one of us is wrong, either us or Indiana, and I hope it's not us, that's all I'm saying.

Dr. Smith: Can I say something?

Mr. Devine: Dr. Smith.

Dr. Smith: From the information that I have, and you can correct me if I'm wrong, I understand that the Public Health authorities thought it was safe in Indiana and the superintendent made the decision against their advice.

Dr. Grady: That is correct. There is no difference between the Indiana Department of Public Health and the Massachusetts Department of Public Health.

Speaker: I'm quoting *TIME* magazine.

Dr. Grady: I know, but I hate to tell you that I have had a little problem with that.

Mr. Devine: Further questions? All right, I don't see any new hands, Mrs. B_____.

Speaker: Thank you. I'd like to know how long are families

of the AIDS victims monitored even after a person who has
AIDS has passed away?

Dr. Grady: You mean in case there was some transmission
in the family, you mean by the request of the family members
themselves because they are concerned, or by a public health
department?

Speaker: Either, it doesn't matter.

Dr. Grady: OK, first of all I want to clarify one thing about
transmission in families. As I said, there has been no instance
of child-to-child transmission. In fact, the children who have
AIDS in some cases get it specifically from their mothers and
at birth. That is the most common cause of transmission. A
typical situation, although by no means the only one, would
be that the mother is a prostitute who uses intravenous drugs
and contracted the disease through contaminated needles—
which makes for a very sad social situation, it's not a healthy
family thing, and now we have the child brought into the world
who's infected. That is the most common source of infection
in children. And by definition, that's mother-to-child, or relative-
to-relative. But that's unique. That's my point, not child-to-
child. The other situations in which children get it are through
the blood transfusions and transfusion products. And that's es-
sentially it. As far as monitoring people, family members have
been looked at because of the social situations that I described.
And sometimes other sex partners, the spouse, or whatever,
have been shown to get it, but through the needle and sexual
contact route later. And I think the longest follow-up studies
now are about three to four years. And transmission has been
shown to take place when those exceptional risk factors are
present, but only then.

Speaker: Thank you.

Mr. Devine: Ma'am, did you have your hand up?

Speaker: Yes, my name is Nadine B——— from Swansea and
I have a daughter in the eighth grade. My question is directed
to you, Mr. Devine. Do you feel there is going to be a problem
with this boy coming back into this school, amongst the students themselves, not as far as the parents, but with the students themselves?

Mr. Devine: The students have been absolutely magnificent

in this entire process. The students who have spoken to me have spoken very positively. They've attempted to articulate some very deep kinds of feelings that they're suddenly becoming aware of, which is also a characteristic of the age level. They're very protective toward their stricken classmate. And again, those students who have expressed their feelings to me are very, very supportive. And I think that they would go to extremes in order to make the youngster feel as comfortable as it would be possible to make him feel under these extremely difficult circumstances.

Speaker: Would you consider having an assembly? My daughter said to me before I came tonight, she said, "Ma, why are you going to the meeting? I think that we should be told, we're the ones that are dealing with it. We're in school with the student all day." Not that she has anything against it because she feels bad and she likes the kid and she wants the kid to come back, like all the other children that I have talked to, they all want him to come back, you know. But they want to know, they want to understand more about it because they're scared just like many of the parents here tonight were.

Mr. Devine: Well, your daughter is a very sensible kid, as are most of her classmates. What we've been doing is, we've been attempting to deal with this as the situation arises, within the classroom setting. I don't think it would be wise to call a large assembly and attempt to explore this kind of topic with a junior high school audience in a large assembly atmosphere. I think that will be counterproductive. But we'll continue to deal with it as the questions arise in class. And hopefully this will satisfy the kids. If they raise a question, they want an answer. They don't want a big, long explanation. They just want an answer that will satisfy them. And this is what the teachers are doing.

Speaker: So they can go to the teachers?

Mr. Devine: Oh absolutely. They can raise a question right in class and that's how we're handling it. Further questions? Yes, in the back.

Speaker: Mr. Devine, I apologize, I am not a resident of Swansea, but I do have a question and I'd like to have permission to ask it of the superintendent who gave me permission to attend and listen this evening.

Mr. Devine: Go ahead, sir.

Speaker: The question is only directed to me as a state official.

Mr. Devine: Excuse me, (*said in a laughing way*) who are you?

Speaker: My name is Philip Travis. I am the state representative for the town of Swansea in the legislature. But I live in the town of Rehoboth, although I have attended Case Junior High School and High School.

Mr. Devine: Thank you, Representative Travis.

Speaker: My question is that there are some people here in truth and conscience who have made a decision that they will not allow their children to attend Case Junior High School. That presents a problem for myself and my office because eventually those people may come to me for assistance. I would like to ask the officer from the state school department and the superintendent, Mr. McCarthy, how will that problem be handled? Are they in violation of state law? Or are there alternatives available if they decide to take that alternative? I would suspect that it will be a very minimum number, from what I've heard, but it is something that may be reality. Thank you.

Mr. Devine: Mr. Hall.

Mr. Hall: The parents who choose to not send their children to a public school, but individually accept the responsibility for placing their children in any approved school, are not in any violation of state law. And that's a decision that all parents have always had the right to do. If, in fact, the question is would the Commonwealth of Massachusetts reimburse the community or directly pay for the educational services of parents who seek educational alternatives, there is no precedent for such payment. And I'm not authorized to indicate that the Department of Education would in any way support funds to the town of Swansea to pay for those services. It's impossible for me to predict what the future would bring in terms of the wishes of the General Court or any other kind of matter. But given current law, such a decision would be a parental decision, the right for them to send their child to an approved school is theirs. The right to receive public monies to do that does not at the present time exist.

Mr. Devine: Mr. McCarthy.

Mr. McCarthy: Representative Travis, I don't know how I can further add to that except to say that if indeed that is the situation, we'll have to deal with that in the future. And I think you've heard the answer from the state Department of Education. I mean you have a right to go to another school if you want to. But not to go to any school is a different kind of an issue.

Mr. Devine: Representative Travis, we certainly have the responsibility to continue to try to work with parents who are still apprehensive—we will! And we will continue to try to find ways to reassure them, just as we have been reassured. I would hope that the door will not slam shut on either side. Further questions? Sir.

Speaker: My question is to you, Mr. Devine. You have mentioned that you would treat every child on an "as need basis" on the information that they need. Junior high and high school is where these children become sexually active, usually. We hope not, of course, but I mean reality is reality. Wouldn't it be better to be forewarned and have them have all the knowledge up front. And wouldn't this be a perfect forum to get all this information out? If you wait for the child to come up with the question, maybe he or she is embarrassed to ask the question. And maybe we should get all this information out beforehand. And on the same token, as I was talking to Mr. McCarthy earlier, maybe this type of a forum should have been done before school started. Let us know that the kid is there. Give us all this information. I for one feel a lot better knowing what we now know from these doctors than before coming here. And so we went for two weeks worried about what was actually going to happen, and you know I feel that getting the information to us, and letting us make the decision, I mean, we are intelligent people, and we should be treated as such and the same with our children.

Mr. Devine: I agree with you. What you are raising is a basic curriculum issue. This topic will certainly become a part of the curriculum. We haven't yet addressed exactly how it's going to be treated, that's why we've been treating it on a need-to-know basis as the situations arise. But you can be assured that the whole subject of AIDS within the larger framework of diseases and disease control, and our knowledge of it as being our best protection, is going to find its way very, very quickly into the junior high school curriculum. It's a curriculum question, and we will be addressing it. We haven't done it yet.

Speaker: What good does it do now? Why didn't you do this before? The kids should have known how to deal with this child.

Mr. Devine: OK, but we received our knowledge, you have to understand, and this was mentioned earlier, that we received our primary knowledge one day before school opened. So we haven't had a whole lot of time to do quality type of curriculum work. This is going to be done, you can be assured of it. Further questions? Ma'am.

Speaker: Sandy P———, I have a daughter in the eighth grade. She came home very upset about this boy, all right. Her concerns were peer pressure, what he was going through. She wanted me to send letters to get him back in school. I'm here tonight, I'm comfortable with what I hear. I love my daughter also. She will be in school. We all have concerns about things that can kill our kids. Yet, where were all these people when they had educational programs for parents on drugs that kill children also? (*applause*)

Mr. Devine: Thank you. I don't see any more hands in the air right now and seeing none, I will take this opportunity to thank our distinguished panel. I really appreciate and I know we all appreciate what they've done for us tonight. (*applause*) And thank you all very much, you've been absolutely magnificent. It's a pleasure being associated with the Swansea schools.

4

*"The kids have really rallied around him.
I'm not afraid because I know I can't
get it (AIDS) just by being his friend. He's not
in school right now because of an ankle
injury, but we all want him back, real soon."*

—Lisa Desnoyers, a classmate

The meeting was over. It had been a very difficult night for me. I had mixed emotions as the crowd filed out of the auditorium. I was glad that my family had chosen not to be interviewed. I'm sure if we had spoken to the press our pictures would have been on front pages across the area. This way, by not being interviewed, I had been able to just walk right into the meeting without being recognized. This is what Dale and I had decided all along. We wanted to be able to go to the Swansea Mall or any place in the area without everyone staring at us and saying "that's the family."

I was extremely pleased with the panel. Everyone on it had done a wonderful job. Mr. Devine, as the moderator, had the responsibility to control the crowd. It was not an easy task because it was such an emotional issue, but Mr. Devine did an excellent job. Mr. McCarthy proved to be a tough administrator. Many people had questioned his decision and he stuck to his judgment. He also showed that he is a very compassionate man and a man who can be trusted. I gained a great deal of knowledge about AIDS by listening to the two doctors. Dr. Smith and Dr. Grady were well prepared for the meeting and it was a pleasure listening to them. Mr. Hall was also well spoken, but I felt bad for him because not too many questions were directed to him.

I suspect that it is not difficult to understand how I felt at that meeting. All the people, all the cameras and equipment, were there because of my son. It seemed like a bad dream. It didn't seem possible that all this was happening. This "afflicted boy" was my son!

People were frightened. You could sense it and I tried to put myself in their place to understand their thoughts and fears. But why weren't they listening to the doctors? AIDS is not spread by casual contact. But time after time, questions and comments dealt with casual contact. It was as if some people never heard what the doctors had said. Right after the doctors would finish an answer about casual contact, the next speaker would be right back with almost the same question. It was very frustrating to me and it must have also been frustrating to the doctors.

I was on an emotional roller coaster. One speaker would raise my spirits by saying good things about Mark, and then the next speaker would have me down in the valley thinking, how can they talk that way about my Mark?

The whole night was like a tennis match with my emotions bouncing back and forth. This was a fellow human being they were talking about—my son! He was a nice kid, well behaved with straight A's in conduct. He was quiet and friendly. He especially loved animals. He was not a threat to anyone. He was very responsible and a tremendous help around the house. He could make mistakes, like everyone else, but he had the unnatural ability to admit them and really be sorry and mean it. If only the parents knew Mark, like the kids in school did, they would have felt much better. He was just a likeable, handsome kid—the girls all loved his extremely long eyelashes.

On the whole, I thought the meeting went well, especially the second half. I thought that many people had been convinced by the doctors. The applause more than the questions revealed how most of the audience felt.

Outside in the parking lot, I saw Dr. Smith walking toward his car. I ran ahead to talk to him and tell him how pleased I was with his presentation. Little did I know that I would be on the phone with him that very night.

Dale's mom had brought Dale and Mark home. Mark was in a lot of pain with his ankle. He had stretched out on the family room rug in front of the TV. He was on Demerol, but it wasn't doing any good. He had Dale rub his ankle but that hurt. He had her pray—to everyone! He was in so much pain!

When I arrived home, I could see a big change in Mark. The pain had increased tremendously. He couldn't even move his leg without terrible agony. I wished that some of the people at that meeting could have seen him then. His inflamed ankle would have certainly brought out some compassion.

I phoned Dr. Smith's house and left word with his son to have him call me as soon as he arrived. A few minutes later the phone rang and it was Dr. Smith. After explaining the situation to him, he told me to give him some more Demerol and to bring Mark to the hospital in the morning. He would call the hospital and make all the arrangements. I told him that he'd better call right away because Mark really needed to go in that night. Dr. Smith agreed and told me to bring him to Rhode Island Hospital in Providence and to use the emergency entrance.

Mark was lying in our bed at the time and he couldn't move. So we decided to call the Swansea ambulance. It seemed to be taking too long, so Dale called again. We also called Dale's mother, who only lives two minutes away, to stay with Scott. The ambulance finally came.

My brother Jeff and his wife Anne came over from their house across the street when they saw the flashing ambulance beacon in our yard.

The young attendant knew about the AIDS case in Swansea and pretty much guessed it was Mark. He didn't know how to ask Dale, he kept hinting until she said, "Yes, Mark has AIDS." She assured him that Mark was not bleeding anywhere. Both EMT's were very nice to Mark. They didn't wear gloves or masks to make Mark feel like a leper. They carefully put Mark on a stretcher since every movement of his body caused his ankle to ache more. Then they wheeled him out of the house. Dale rode in the ambulance with Mark and I followed in our little red '84 Aries. Dale said that Mark would cry out in pain every time they went over a bump.

It was another new experience for me to follow an ambulance at speeds of about 90 M.P.H. down I-195. I wasn't even sure if the car could go that fast. But I wanted to keep up because I knew how scared Mark was and I wanted to be able to help comfort him. We were at the hospital in no time and, since it was late at night, I found a parking space right away. I joined

Mark and Dale as the attendants were wheeling Mark into the hospital.

The nurses asked a few questions and then someone led us to the Potter Wing—the pediatric section. I learned that Mark would be staying on the first floor which is the teenage section. Other floors are for different age groups. I'm glad the person guiding us knew where to go because it seemed like we walked for a mile through countless tunnels and corridors. It was like a dungeon. The first floor corridor, where Mark would stay, was very dark and frightening to me. We had been in sections of Rhode Island Hospital before when the boys came for check-ups with Dr. Smith, but we had never been in the emergency room there, or been on this floor in this particular building. Mark had never stayed at Rhode Island Hospital in Providence. Little did we know at the time that the Potter Building would be a second home for us all.

There were two female residents on duty that night and a very pleasant nurse. All that was done for Mark that night was to give him some pain medication through an IV. He didn't really sleep the rest of the night and we didn't either.

The next morning there were blood tests and an orthopedic doctor came in to see Mark. I was really impressed that the doctors and nurses didn't wear gowns and masks like they did at St. Anne's Hospital.

The young orthopedic doctor came in to see Mark and scared Dale by what he had to say. He thought that it was probably some type of infection and Mark would probably need an operation. But, first, he would have to drain the ankle to see what was inside.

Dale did not want to stay in the room while the doctor drained Mark's ankle. She doesn't like things like that for one thing and, secondly, the room was very small. Mark had liked his large suite at St. Anne's Hospital but this room was more like a prison cell. The room was only about eight feet across and maybe 12 feet long. The bed and a small sink were on the left side and two small chairs and a bureau were on the right side. The bathroom was diagonally across the hall from his room.

The orthopedic doctor and a nurse came in. I stood behind Mark, at the head of the bed, and held both his hands. First,

he explained everything to Mark. Mark wanted to know if it
would hurt and he said it probably would. Then the doctor put
a needle right into Mark's ankle to freeze it. Mark squeezed my
hands tightly, but he kept his ankle very still. It really killed
him. I could tell it hurt him and felt so bad for him. Then the
doctor took another large needle and a syringe and stuck it into
the ankle. Mark yelled out in pain and squeezed my hands even
tighter than before. But he still didn't move! He was one brave
kid! And he had a talent for putting himself into a trance when
he used to get his needles at Pediatrics in Fall River. We practically lived there until Mark was about 10. And all the doctors
were impressed with Mark and how still he could stay.

When the doctor drew on the syringe, a sickening yellow
fluid filled it. He used another needle and syringe, again Mark
yelled in pain, and again more yellow fluid came out. It was
definitely an infection because the doctor had said that if blood
came out it was probably just a bad bleed. It turned out to be
salmonella that had been circulating in his bloodstream and
found its way to Mark's weakest point, which at that time was
the right ankle. The doctors decided that they would have to
operate to get all of the infection out.

The operation was scheduled for later that afternoon. Mark
wouldn't be able to drink or eat for the rest of the day. I had
to call into work to tell Sister Martha that I wouldn't be in. Dr.
Phillip Lucas, a very pleasant doctor, who Dale thought was
very handsome, would do the surgery. He came to see Mark
and us and we all liked him right away.

Once again, for the second time, we would accompany our
son to the operating room. This time, the walk was much longer
than the walk at St. Anne's. Once again we would get to a door
that said No Admittance Beyond This Point, and we would
both kiss Mark and wish him good luck. We decided to go to
a floor with vending machines and couches so we could sit and
try to relax a bit. My sister and mother came up to keep us company. I bought a couple of papers to see what they would say
about last night's meeting. I later learned that all the TV stations had the meeting as their feature story. But we did not see
any of them.

The front page of the *Providence Journal-Bulletin* had a large
picture of Lenny C——— with the quote, "You ain't going to

leave a kid going around with a gallon of gas and a match, that's how I see it," under his picture, which also showed a section of the auditorium and the large crowd. The September 12 paper had a headline: "500 hear experts on AIDS; many fears are not relieved." The front page also had smaller pictures of Superintendent John McCarthy and Dr. Peter Smith. Another page had a picture of the four panelists: Dr. Smith, Dr. Grady, Mr. Hall, and Superintendent McCarthy.

The story by Irene Wielawski with reports from Linda Borg, Bob Jagolinzer, W. Malinowski, and Jody McPhillips talked about the depth of the anguish of the people of Swansea. It went on to give some quotes from the meeting by individual speakers.

"Several parents leaving the meeting said they felt reassured by the meeting. Some said they were still scared and upset. Others said they needed time to think over all that was said during the emotional, three-hour session."

Later in the article it said: "The boy's name, while widely known in this close-knit community of 15,000, has been zealously guarded by school officials, doctors involved in the case and, last night, by even those most vehement in their opposition to his presence in school. The boy, his parents, and younger brother did not attend last night's meeting."

The article also talked about Dr. Smith's week. "Smith has been deluged with requests for interviews by the newspapers around the country, by television networks and radio talk show hosts."

Dr. Smith described his feelings after the meeting as being "exhausted." He thought the majority of the people were there just to listen. "Just to take this all in. They need time to let it sink in, argue about it."

The *Fall River Herald-News* had similar front page pictures. They had a picture of Lenny C———, Dr. Smith, and Superintendent McCarthy. Their heading was: "Swansea parents told AIDS risk 'zero.'" Fred Rhines in his report said, "Two medical experts Wednesday night advised nearly 600 parents of students at Joseph Case Junior High School, in Swansea, that an AIDS-stricken 8th grade student attending that school poses no risk to other students."

The article went on to give quotes of the panelists and to

talk about the way the discussion went on for more than three hours in a "see-sawed, back and forth" manner. Then it gave quotes from some of the speakers and Reggie Desnoyers' daughter. Lisa said that she "played hide-and-seek with the stricken boy just the other day." She added, "The kids have really rallied around him. I'm not afraid because I know I can't get it (AIDS) just by being his friend. He's not in school right now because of an ankle injury, but we all want him back, real soon."

The weekly newspaper *The Spectator* had the heading: "Meeting eases anxiety about AIDS situation." A subheading said: "Transmission risk termed 'zero.'"

The story by Cheryl Crossley-O'Brien mentioned that "the townspeople have predominantly rallied to the support of the action of Superintendent John McCarthy in his decision in allowing the youngster to participate in the regular school day." She went on like the other reporters to talk about the questions asked and the responses of the panel. At the end of her article, she called Mark an "unwilling pioneer."

Mark Patinkin, a syndicated columnist for the *Providence Journal,* wrote a heartwarming article about Swansea. The title was: "A child's plight brought out the very best in a small town." He wrote about the number of children with AIDS who had been barred from school and the number of boycotts held. But one place seemed different to him — Swansea, Massachusetts. He discussed cases in Indiana and New York and then the Swansea meeting that he attended. He quoted parents and Superintendent McCarthy, whom he did not envy, because to quote Patinkin: "What do you say to 600 people who feel you've jeopardized their children?" When McCarthy was finished explaining his decision, "That is when an unexpected thing happened. His answer drew the loudest applause I'd heard so far.

"And that is how it went. Two thirds of those who spoke were skeptics, but I suppose that is human nature. The angry speak up more often. The sentiment of the majority, however, stood loudest behind those who called for fairness for this one, stricken child."

Mr. Patinkin went on talking about an interview he had with the Case Junior High principal and how Mr. Devine had said that Swansea had "a willingness to become informed before making judgments." Mr. Patinkin closed with, "I had not expected to hear that message. I think it's something I will remember—that in this one place, on this most difficult of issues, the voices of emotion were drowned out by the voices of reason."

You could never know how happy this article made my entire family feel. It was great to know that an outsider felt the same way as I did about that meeting—the majority were behind Mr. McCarthy's decision to allow Mark in school. This type of article was just what we needed, something positive for a change.

Dale, Jayne, my mom, and I walked back to Mark's room because we wanted to be there when they brought him back. Nancy Keyes and Debbie DeMaio (nurse and social worker) were already there waiting for us. These two young women helped our family tremendously through all the tough times. They were not just professionals doing their jobs, they were good friends!

Finally, Dr. Lucas came by to tell us that everything went well and that Mark was in the recovery room and would be down soon.

We continued to talk about Mark and his positive attitude. He really had his mind set on beating this disease. Every day he would give me the thumbs up sign which meant "I'm going to win." He talked about AIDS a great deal with me, but he never mentioned it to any of his friends as far as I know. In fact, he hardly talked about it with anyone except me. He just went on living life day by day and making the most of it. Looking at him you would never know he had AIDS. He had gained back the weight he had lost and looked good. If it wasn't for that damn ankle, things would be pretty normal in his life—if living with AIDS can be considered normal. Well, maybe it was best that he wasn't in school at that time. How would he be able to face all that publicity? In a way, I was glad that he didn't have to. Why did all this have to be in the newspapers anyway? Mark was going to school and minding his own business and everything was fine. Life certainly can be challenging!

Mark was wheeled into the room and gently transferred to

his bed. The anesthesiologist said he had done wonderfully. The ankle was all bandaged up and Mark was only partially conscious. He did say hi and a few other things before he dozed off again. Later, when he woke up he was very thirsty. He talked to all of us.

Mark liked the Potter Building. There were many young nurses and Mark seemed to hit it off well with all of them. Probably Pam Cote was his favorite. She was blond and unmarried. They were always joking with each other. She always wore a smile and Mark's face seemed to brighten when she was around. Mark also liked the snacks in Potter I. And they were available anytime at all—day or night. They had juices and punches and soda and ice cream and all the "goodies" a teenager would want. The nurses would get them, but since Dale and I were there all the time, we waited on him ourselves. They had a VCR hooked up to a color TV that could be brought into the room. Each week they rented new movies and they always had a good selection. There were other activities going on during the week and creative projects that could be done without having to leave the bed. They also had special days such as Italian Day. Every week a specially designed cart would stop by and the patients could pick their favorite Italian food. Mark loved Italian food, so this was one of his favorite days. Another day the treat was to make your own sundae. The food was probably about the same as the other hospital, but to Mark it was a change and so it seemed better to him. At the end of the hall there was a teen center where parents were not allowed. It had video games, a TV, "Atari," a phone, board games, activity items, couches and chairs, and so forth. Mark liked this room, too.

I had taken Thursday, September 12, off from school and I also missed a meeting I was supposed to go to on Friday. So this gave me four days to spend at the hospital counting the weekend. Dale and I rotated sleeping at the hospital again while the other went home with Scott. One good thing about Rhode Island Hospital was that they let family members in to visit. So Scott could also come up after school and stay until one of us went home with him. At least we were all together as a family.

Mark had many visitors as usual. My parents, Dale's parents, my sister and brothers and their families, Dale's brother and his family, and other friends. He also received many cards which he hung on his door. Friends bought him posters and decorations that he put on the walls. We also had our own little store of goodies from home.

The ankle was still bothering Mark and they kept him hooked up to the IV machine for pain medication, factor VIII, and chlorophenical, which was to fight the salmonella.

As soon as he was able, they started him on light therapy with Susan Gemma, his hemophilia therapist. We had known Sue from our yearly checkups, but we became much closer seeing her on a daily basis in the hospital and later when she would come to our house twice a week for 10 months. Mark and Sue became good friends eventually, but at first he hated to see her come because the therapy pained him so much.

The newspapers also found out Mark was in the hospital. The *Fall River Herald-News* had the headline: "Injury hospitalizes young AIDS victim." The article, written by Fred Rhines, told how he was in satisfactory condition at Rhode Island Hospital, having been admitted the same night as the Swansea meeting. It went on to tell what Dr. Smith had said about the boy and then went into the school situation and how Mr. Devine "stated attendance was 'better than 94 percent' Thursday morning following the informational meeting, and he added, 'In fact, attendance was a little better than it had been before the meeting.'" This was encouraging to read.

The *Providence Journal* had the headline: "Swansea AIDS victim admitted to hospital." A subheading said: "8th-grader suffers from hemophilia complications."

It seemed like every day that we were at the hospital there would be an article in one of the newspapers about Mark. And many people were writing editorials and letters to the editor about Mark and Superintendent McCarthy.

A survey done by the *Herald-News* at Swansea Mall entitled, "Most favor letting AIDS student continue his regular schooling," gave opinions of people interviewed there. The headline says it all.

The *Spectator* had a couple of items about Mark under the general heading: "Support for student grows." The subheadings were: "Rep. Frank affirms government support, commends McCarthy" and "Classmates, parents, teachers rally." Congressional Representative Barney Frank praised McCarthy when he spoke with reporter Cheryl Crossley-O'Brien. "I think Superintendent McCarthy really distinguished himself in a responsible and courageous way. . . . He read up on it and determined there is in fact no danger. . . . He's very respectful of the rights of others. I admire him in this regard."

The other article written by Barbara Davies stated: "Following the example of the Swansea school administration, the children, their parents and teachers of the Joseph Case Junior High, along with many town residents are rallying in support of a student who is a victim of AIDS. The students of the junior high are discussing finding a way to work for financial support to further medical research for a cure of this virus."

Stories like these made our day and helped Mark very much. He had read all about Ryan White in Indiana, another young hemophiliac who contracted AIDS through the blood treatments. And he had seen on TV how the people in Kokomo treated Ryan. I know he felt bad for him and I'm sure he must have feared the same thing happening to him. But Swansea was turning out to be the town with compassion and we all welcomed this good fortune.

Other good stories appeared across Massachusetts. "AIDS boy's pals: We want to help" read the headline in the *Boston Herald*. Gayle Fee wrote about the 15 students who approached Mr. Devine before school one morning with plans for a community fundraising drive. "Devine said he and school Superintendent John E. McCarthy received a number of calls and letters from parents praising their decision to let the eighth-grader with AIDS attend classes. 'I think we've weathered the initial storm,' said Devine. 'Kids, being kids, are now pursuing how they can help this victim. They are anxious to become active in some sort of activity that will be of some direct help to this youngster. Parents have expressed the same kind of concerns. . . . The support has been great.'"

The editor of the *Herald* in Boston also supported the Swansea decision and so did the *Boston Globe*. Another article that came out when Mark was in the hospital was written by Zachary Malinowski. In the *Evening-Bulletin*, the headline was: "AIDS victim's friends are many, loyal, vocal." The subheadline said: "Baseball coach, classmates stand by the youth, remind that he is in many ways a normal teen." The morning edition of the *Providence Journal* had basically the same story with Reggie Desnoyers' picture. The headline was: "AIDS victim's friends remind public at issue's heart is normal boy, his family."

The story told how Reggie sneaked into the hospital with coach Leo Roy to visit Mark at St. Anne's. Reggie talked about Mark being a "standout on the Swansea Giants for the past three years. If not for the AIDS virus, which forced the boy to miss eight games, he would have been a shoo-in for the All-Star team." In fact, Reggie went on to say that he had been "coaching for 17 years, and he (Mark) rates in the top 10 or 12 players during that time."

Jody Donnelly was also interviewed and she talked about her son Shane being best friends with Scott. Of course, Scott's name wasn't mentioned. She told the *Journal* how Shane was always at our house, and how both Mark and Scott had been to her house many times. Mark was a good friend with her oldest son, Todd. She described Mark as a "fantastic athlete. Both boys are. They are normal, active boys."

Jody also mentioned the banner that the students at Case Junior made for Mark. It had little messages from over a hundred students. Mark enjoyed reading them and hung them across the wall over his bed. He also received many cards and letters from the students at my school, St. John's.

One letter to the editor that appeared in the *Journal-Bulletin* brought back a haunting question. Who told the newspapers about Mark? The letter was written by a doctor from Swansea who said he was outraged as a physician over the issue of confidentiality. His letter concerned the September 5 front page article. Quoting Dr. Leffer, "The article states that Swansea 'teachers anonymously contacted the *Journal-Bulletin*' because of their concerns. One can only assume that the only effects they had hoped to gain by contacting a newspaper would be to create enough negative publicity to hound this courageous young boy out of the school system. The teachers should feel great shame in betraying the confidentiality of this student in the manner they chose. Their fears may certainly be real, but they showed a deplorable insensitivity in how they let them be known."

More and more letters to the editor were being sent to various newspapers supporting Mark. And other newspapers in Boston, New Bedford, and Attleboro had articles about Mark. Robert Lecomte, whose daughter was in the seventh grade at Case Junior, speaking to Philip Bennett of the *Boston Globe* said, "When the news came out, it was spoken about in the corner stores, everywhere, and it really went through the community like wildfire. But people here are thinking with their hearts. The consensus is, why deprive this child of an education? All the children feel really strongly about it, and I haven't heard a complaint from any of the parents I've spoken with."

Newsday in New York had an article about Mark with pictures of Mr. McCarthy and Reggie Desnoyers. The *New York Times* also had a story about Swansea. The *New Bedford Standard Times* in an editorial supported Mr. McCarthy. Most newspapers did, but there were some people who were not convinced.

One of these people was Mrs. Terese Fagundes of Swansea. She talked about starting a petition to keep Mark out of school at the meeting and she certainly did try. The *Fall River Herald-News* on Thursday, September 19, had her picture and an article about her. We were informed of this beforehand by an anonymous tip from somebody who lived on her street. It made us feel terrible. My brother Jeff was so angry that he drove down to the Little League field where she was stationed and got into a heated debate with her. My parents also drove down there, but just sat in the car each night from a distance to see whether anyone would sign. Dale and I were upset, it certainly didn't make us feel very good, but we just didn't let it bother us like it did my brother and parents. However, the fact that she picked the Little League Field did bother us a bit.

Mrs. Fagundes said she would be on the field for three days. "I wish I didn't have to do what I'm doing," she stated to Fred Rhines, a *Herald-News* reporter. "The boy is certainly entitled to an education. I'm doing it because of the risk involved to others. The school department is not stopping the child from having contact with others."

On Wednesday night she had eight signatures. She claimed to get 23 from her neighborhood on Sharps Lot Road. I was told many of these people didn't even have children at the school, but signed it as a favor to their neighbor.

The next night she had five more signatures. The *Journal* article told how "she got into an argument with a man who identified himself as a relative of the sick child. While Mrs. Fagundes was collecting signatures a man walked up to her and said, 'I think what you are doing is atrocious!' He also complained that Mrs. Fagundes was refusing to listen to medical experts who have said there is no danger that other children in the school would get AIDS from the stricken child. He asserted that Mrs. Fagundes was leading the petition drive 'for publicity.'" (The unidentified man was my brother Jeff.)

Mrs. Fagundes, who has two daughters at the junior high school, said that she had "every right to collect the signatures." My brother left after getting in a few more choice sentences.

But there were others whose minds and hearts told them to stand by this boy.

A "N.A. mother" (North Attleboro) wrote an anonymous letter to the editor in an Attleboro paper:

> I am writing in regard to that poor boy in Swansea who has AIDS. I don't know how people can be so cruel.
>
> This boy has to deal first of all with his blood disorder. Something he has to live in fear with. Then he finds out he has AIDS. Now he has two horrible diseases he has to deal with, one a definite killer in the near future.
>
> But he must find the courage to deal with it because he decides to try to live a near as possible "normal life." He decides to keep going to school instead of saying, 'hey, screw it. I'm going to die anyway. Why don't I stay home and live it up.'
>
> But no, he wants to continue his education and he gets pushed down. I can imagine how he must feel, living with his blood disease, living with AIDS, and living as if he was a piece of nothing because people are condemning him for circumstances beyond his control.
>
> This child is not a baby that puts toys in his mouth and parents are afraid their children will put the same toys in their mouth. That concern I can understand. But this boy is in junior high. He has been told I'm sure about precautions.
>
> People are lashing out because of the fear they have from the unknown. But there is enough evidence that AIDS is not transmitted casually. You people should be

happy this person knows he has AIDS and knows how to protect other people.

I think he and other children of AIDS need the support of their peers. They need a reason to want to fight to live. The will to live is a big part of surviving with so many ill-nesses. You need that strength.

I think if you want to be afraid of something be afraid of how many people have AIDS without the signs as the carriers of AIDS. How many public places do you go — stores, restaurants, church, clubs, work, movies, etc.— and people cough, sneeze, talk; and how do you know if that person has AIDS? Are you going to refrain from all social activity because of AIDS?

I think you should have more fear for the people who don't know they have AIDS and are transmitting it rather than someone who knows they have it and can protect others. Your own child could have sex with a person who has AIDS or even other family members. Would you want them to be condemned or understood?

The last I read he was in the hospital because of his blood disease.

Does that make everyone happy because he is now out of the way? If it does you are sicker than he is!

To anyone who has AIDS: Please don't think too badly on the people that fear you. Remember it's not you per-sonally but the fear of not knowing this disease.

I'm scared. I have children, some of which are dating, and even though they know about AIDS I hope they are careful so they don't catch it. But if they did I would give them my support and I hope others would and that's why I cannot condemn anyone else because you never know when it can happen to you or someone you love.

And would you turn your back on them, or would you want everyone to turn their back on you?

I hope they find a cure for AIDS fast because if people are getting in an uproar about one person, I'd hate to see what's going to happen when the number of people with AIDS keeps doubling.

People will probably be afraid to leave their houses.

5

"One night the Town of Swansea turned the lights on across America."

—Edward J. Durand in the
Fall River Herald-News

Since Mark's salmonella infection was not life threatening as long as it stayed in the ankle, I went back to school on Monday, the 16th. After school, I would drive directly to the hospital, down I-95 from Attleboro. Dale would then take our car home to shower and be there when Scott arrived from school at about 3:45 P.M.

I believe it was Monday, the 16th, when the students in my class started asking me if Mark was the Swansea boy who had been in all the papers. My eighth graders were a very special class and very mature for their age and I spent a whole period during religion class telling them all about Mark and what we had been through since June. I never regretted telling them because I knew they could be trusted and they were very understanding. Later in the year, we started a Human Sexuality curriculum and AIDS was one of the topics covered. Franny Powers and Shelley Gauthier, the seventh and sixth grade homeroom teachers, also did lessons on AIDS. When the students in those grades had questions for me about AIDS, I always took time out of my history classes to answer them. Our Human Sexuality course starts in the first grade and has the backing of all the parents, particularly since we held meetings to explain the program and showed them the slides, movies, and videos that we would be using with the children. I think the program has been a great success and I believe that the children at St. John the Evangelist knew more about AIDS than most students in the country. Of course, the Swansea public schools

117

also did a great job teaching about AIDS. Every school in the country should teach about AIDS.

Mark seemed more comfortable as the days passed but his ankle was still very sore. He would have to be on the chloro-phenical IV for quite some time.

Dr. Smith visited every day and so did Debbie DeMaio, Nancy Keyes, and Sue Gemma. They began to talk about letting Mark go home with an IV machine. Since I knew how to give the treatment and so did Mark, it would be easier on us all if Mark could just go home and recover there. Of course, we would have to learn how to operate the IV pump and keep the saline solu-tion flowing all the time and how to handle little problems that might develop, like air in the tubes, but we thought we could handle it. They told us that there were home care com-panies that could supply us with the IV pole, pump, and every-thing we needed for the medication. However, they would be switching the medication from IV chlorophenical to IV ampi-cillin. Dr. Smith thought the ampicillin would work just as well. He would be on the IV machine for three weeks at home, taking 1.75 grams every six hours. We would have to mix the ampicillin powder with 13.6 cc of sterile water to achieve 125 mg./cc and give 14 cc of IV push as directed by the physician. It all seemed so complicated. But if we could do it, Mark would be able to go home and that is what he – and we – really wanted. A nurse from Home Nutritional Support, Inc. came down to Rhode Island Hospital to show me how to do everything. She would also come to the house the first day to watch us give the medication for the first time. Then we would be on our own.

So on Thursday, September 19, Dale's mother's birthday, Mark came home. He had spent eight days and nights in the hospital. His total hospital stay since coming down with AIDS was now 35 days in three months' time. Dale's mom offered to give Mark a ride home so I wouldn't have to take another day off.

Mark was in a very happy mood when I arrived home. He gave me a big hug and kiss. Nancy Keyes had come down to visit to make sure everything was OK and to hook him back up to the IV machine. She had put a heperon lock on his vein so he could travel freely on the way home. She also showed us how to use a heperon lock so that we could free Mark during the day if he wanted. We went on a schedule of giving the medication at midnight, 6:00 A.M., noontime, and 6:00 P.M. It wasn't easy, but we didn't have any problems until Saturday, the 21st.

We put a heperon lock on Mark and he used his crutches to walk down to his room. With a heperon lock, you still have the IV catheter in your vein, but a clamp shuts off the vein. The vein does not collapse and start to clot because of the heperon solution. Well, Mark wasn't down to his room five minutes when I heard him yell, "Dad, Dad, come here quick! Dad!" I rushed down to his bedroom and found blood gushing out of his arm. It was everywhere! The desk, the rug—just all over. Mark had evidently knocked the needle out of the vein or somehow knocked the clamp. I tried the clamp first, but it didn't stop the bleeding, so it had to be that the needle was loose. The blood kept pouring out and I couldn't stop it. His arm was all bandaged up and it was impossible to see exactly where it was coming from. I tried to get the taped bandages off as quickly as I could. Blood was all over my hands by now, too. Finally, I succeeded in getting the arm unwrapped and taking the needle out. I held his arm with some gauze and the bleeding eventually stopped. We had the worst luck! Dale called our next door neighbor, Rita Brennan, who is a nurse, to come over to comfort Mark and us.

Mark was more calm now, but worried about not being able to be connected to the machine. I said if worse came to worse, I could just give him the ampicillin like I do the factor VIII, by putting a needle into his vein and just pushing the ampicillin through. Of course, I would have had to check with Dr. Smith first.

I called Nancy Keyes at her home and she told me to just use an IV infusion set with the hard needle (rather than the soft catheter needle which is harder to put in) and hook him back up to the machine like that. She would come out Monday morning and put a new catheter in. Mark felt better after hearing this. Needless to say, Mark never tried the heperon lock at home again.

Also on the 21st, Mark's ankle started bothering him again. We thought it was probably a bleed from trying to do too much therapy. We gave him treatment through the IV machine which I had hooked back up.

Sunday and Monday Mark was still having ankle problems.

I gave him treatment each day through the IV machine. At least I didn't have to stick him with a needle. I called Dr. Smith at his home on Sunday and told him about Mark's discomfort. He said he had to go to Swansea that afternoon and would stop by our house. We were all impressed with this. A doctor who would make a house call—and on a Sunday yet! Dr. Smith looked at Mark and said that if it continued to bother him, he would probably have to have it tapped again. In the meantime, we were to continue the factor VIII in case it was a bleed and he gave us a prescription for codeine. No one could ever know how much pain that ankle gave Mark!

On Tuesday and Wednesday the ankle started to get worse again. I gave him double treatments both days through the IV pump. Nancy Harkness came over to visit on Wednesday and Mark was very happy to see her. He loved to have visitors. He acted a little silly that day, the way the kids sometimes acted when they were having a bleed.

I called Dr. Smith and he said the ankle would definitely have to be looked at by Dr. Lucas. We called the office late in the day and got an appointment for the next day. Thursday, Mark was getting extremely uncomfortable again. Dale and I were beginning to think that it might be more infection. We hadn't thought so at first, because he was on the ampicillin. But maybe that medicine wasn't working as well as the chloro-phenical did.

On Thursday I did not go to work so I could bring Mark to the doctors. Dr. Lucas took Mark right away even though the waiting room was crowded with patients. This reminded me of the special treatment we had always received from the doctors and nurses at Fall River Pediatrics. They always took us as soon as we walked in the door. Ginny Morrisette was one of the pedi nurses who became a close friend.

Dr. Lucas felt the ankle did need draining again. Mark was afraid of that. He well remembered the terrible pain he had experienced exactly two weeks ago when it was done for the first time. He also remembered the soreness from the bone marrow test which was done by Dr. Smith that same day. Mark didn't mind needles going into his veins, but he did mind needles going into other parts of his body. I hated to see Mark in so much pain and wished that I could suffer it for him.

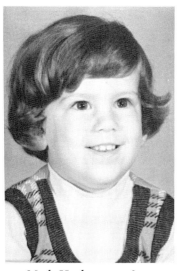

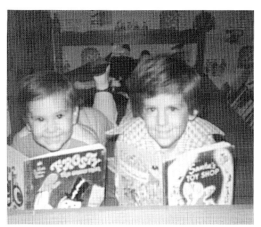

The Hoyle brothers enjoy Christmas 1976—Scott, 1½, on the left; Mark, 4.

Mark Hoyle at age 2—a captivating toddler.

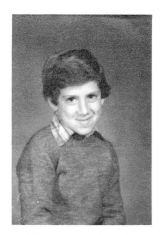

Mark—second grade photo.

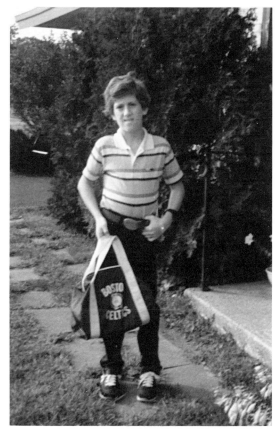

Ready to set off for the first day of school in the fourth grade.

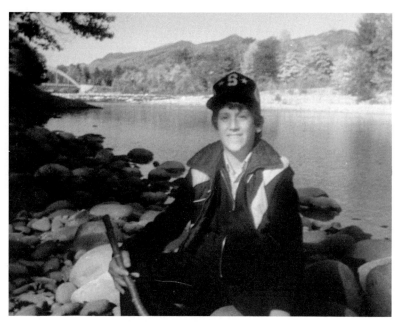

At age 10, in New Hampshire, one of Mark's favorite vacation spots.

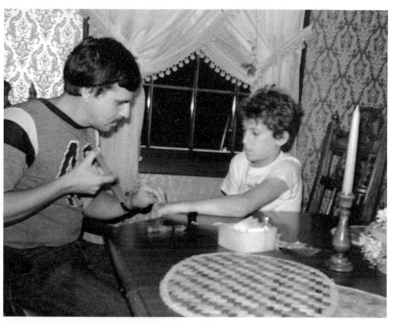

Jay Hoyle administers Mark's factor VIII treatment.

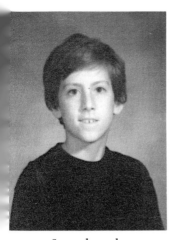

Seventh grade
class photo.

1984: A passion for
baseball—a Red Sox fan
and a star in the
Swansea Little League.

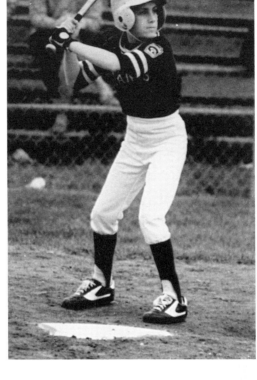

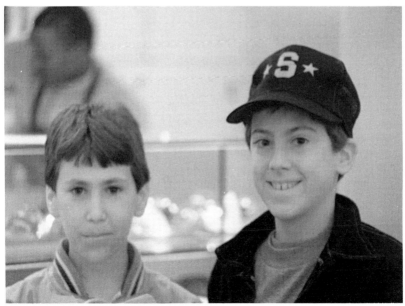

Mark (right) with brother Scott—not just brothers, but best friends as well.

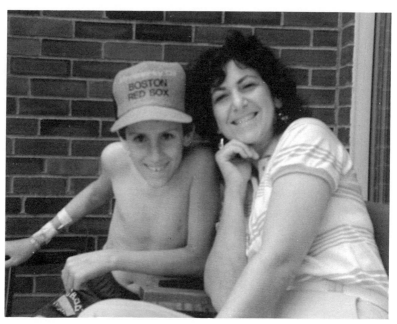

Mark and mom Dale during Mark's July 1985 hospitalization at St. Anne's.

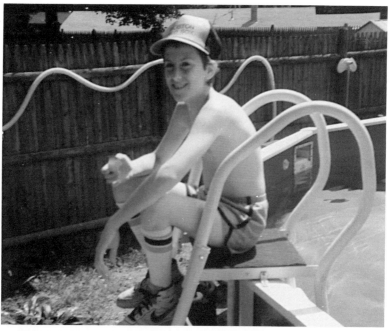

August 1985: Mark enjoys sunning at the Hoyles' backyard pool.

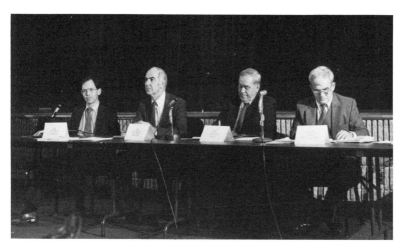

The issue of AIDS is discussed in Swansea, September 11, 1985, at
Case High School. Pictured here, left to right: Dr. Peter Smith,
director of the Hemophilia Center of Rhode Island; Dr. George Grady,
associate state commissioner of the Department of Public Health; Mr.
Curtis Hall, chief of the Department of Education's office in Lakeville,
MA; John E. McCarthy, Swansea school superintendent.

Photograph: Hank Pollard. Courtesy of the *Fall River Herald-News*

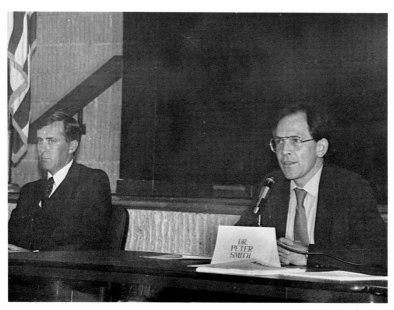

Mr. Harold Devine, principal of Case Junior High School, and Dr.
Peter Smith, Mark's physician, at the Swansea meeting.

Photograph: Hank Pollard. Courtesy of the *Fall River Herald-News*

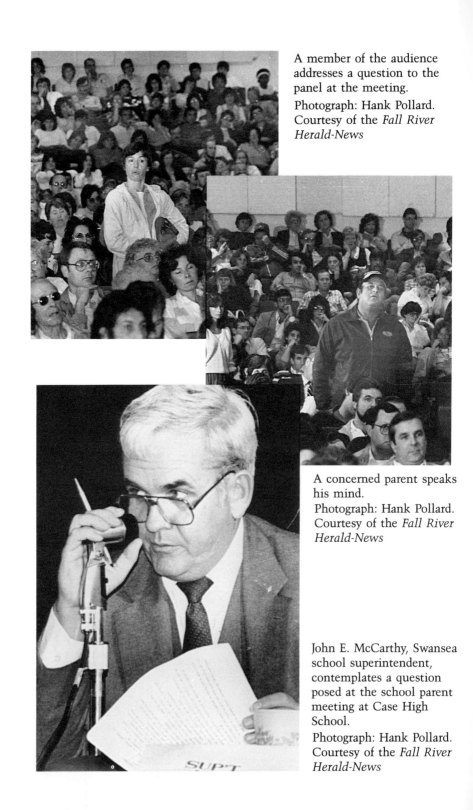

A member of the audience addresses a question to the panel at the meeting.
Photograph: Hank Pollard. Courtesy of the *Fall River Herald-News*

A concerned parent speaks his mind.
Photograph: Hank Pollard. Courtesy of the *Fall River Herald-News*

John E. McCarthy, Swansea school superintendent, contemplates a question posed at the school parent meeting at Case High School.
Photograph: Hank Pollard. Courtesy of the *Fall River Herald-News*

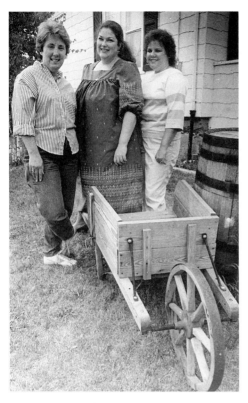

Linda Nahas, Susan Travers, and Robin Sherman. Founders of the "Friends of Mark," these three concerned mothers ignited the spirit of caring and compassion in Swansea.

Photograph: Courtesy of the *New Bedford Standard Times*

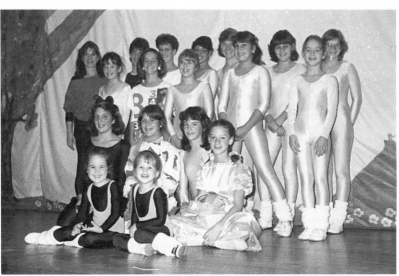

Leading off a series of events planned by the "Friends of Mark" was a performance at Case Junior High School by these creative dance students.

Photograph: Barbara Davies. Courtesy of *The Somerset Spectator*

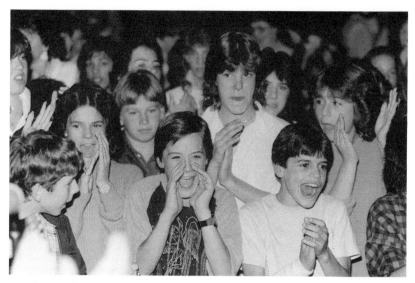

"That's What Friends Are For"—student dance held as a fundraiser for Mark.

Courtesy of the *Providence Journal Company*

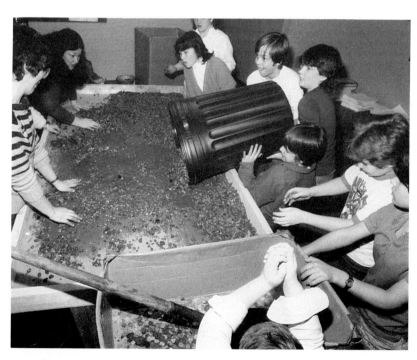

Students sort out coins from the Swansea Mall wishing well. Wishing well coins were donated by the mall to the "Friends of Mark."

Courtesy of the *Providence Journal Company*

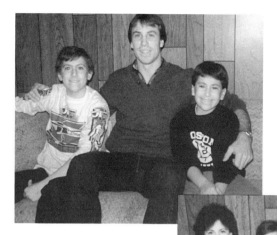

January 1986: Mark and Scott enjoy a visit from their cousin, Greg Gagne, shortstop of the Minnesota Twins.

The Hoyle family in the spring of 1986—Dale, Mark, Scott, and Jay.

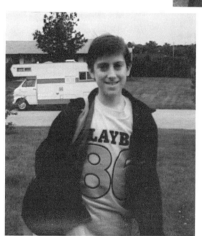

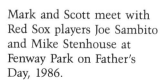

The last day of school, June 1986—Mark received the Principal's Award, presented annually to a deserving boy and girl at Case Junior High School.

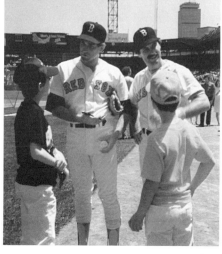

Mark and Scott meet with Red Sox players Joe Sambito and Mike Stenhouse at Fenway Park on Father's Day, 1986.

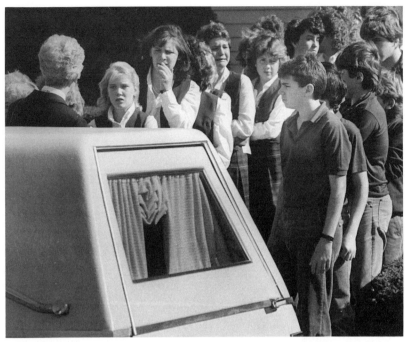

Students from St. John the Evangelist School mourn the loss of their teacher's son.

Photograph: Jack Iddon. Courtesy of the *New Bedford Standard Times*

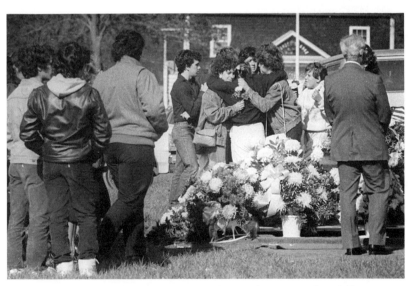

Classmates from Case High School console one another following graveside services for Mark at Mt. Hope Cemetery in Swansea.

Photograph: Jack Iddon. Courtesy of the *New Bedford Standard Times*

"We pray that God takes great care of you for us . . ." At Mt. Hope Cemetery—Jay, Scott, Dale, Mark's cousin Joshua, and Mark's Aunt Anne.

Photograph: Jack Iddon. Courtesy of the *New Bedford Standard Times*

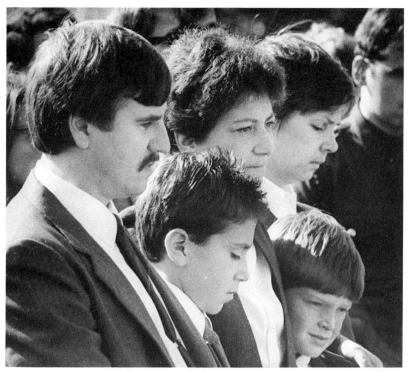

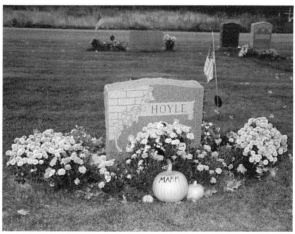

"Remember him, and live for him."

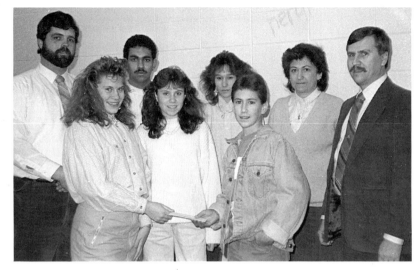

A $1,000 contribution to the Mark Gardiner Hoyle Scholarship Fund is presented by Case High School freshmen, with Scott Hoyle accepting on behalf of the Hoyle family.

Photograph: Barbara Davies. Courtesy of *The Somerset Spectator*

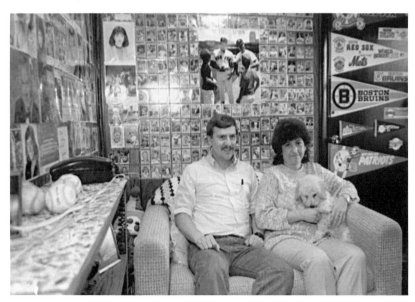

Jay and Dale Hoyle at home in the Sports Room dedicated to Mark.

Dr. Lucas was as gentle as possible. Dale left the room again. I held Mark's hand as the nurse assisted the doctor. I was eager to see the color of the liquid. It came out reddish. This made me happy, it was probably just a bad bleed. But Dr. Lucas said that even though it looked like blood, there could be infection in the blood or in some pocket in the ankle where the needle hadn't reached. Tests would have to be done and this would take a few days. Meanwhile, Mark could go home with a prescription for more pain medication. He would also continue on the ampicillin.

Before he left the house for the doctor's office, I had given Mark an additional two vials of factor VIII and then pulled out the IV. Nancy Keyes met us at Dr. Lucas' office and put in a new IV for Mark with a heperon lock to get us home. As soon as we arrived we hooked Mark back up to the IV pump because he was nervous about the heperon lock.

I watched the Weather Channel because it looked like our area was going to be directly hit by a hurricane with over 200 M.P.H. winds. We hadn't had any real major hurricanes since I was a kid. But I did remember a couple back then, one in particular, Hurricane Carol, which had done a great deal of damage and always stuck in my mind.

This time it was Hurricane Gloria making its way up the Atlantic seaboard. It didn't look good so I decided to call the Electric Light Company to tell them that I needed electricity for an IV pump for Mark. They told me that they would put my street on the list of priorities in case the power went out. This meant, supposedly, that they would work to get the electricity back to our street as soon as possible after it went off. I felt better about this, but not about the approaching hurricane.

School was called off the next day, Friday, September 27, because of the storm. The wind picked up as the morning passed and Mark was still in pain. We were still giving him the ampicillin every six hours and I gave him two more vials of treatment in the morning. Scott, Dale, and I kept looking out the windows and watching the wind blow the trees, but poor Mark couldn't enjoy the excitement. He was just lying on the mattress on the floor of the family room. His arm was hooked up to the machine. It became apparent that we would not get the full force of the storm with its torrential rains, but we could still get some very high winds. And winds we did get! As the three of us looked out the sliding glass doors in the family room, the old dead pine tree (about 70 feet high) in my neighbor's yard came crashing down right in front of our eyes. It knocked down two sections of my six-foot high stockade fence, breaking it into little pieces. It also squashed a small white birch tree I had growing in the yard. It was exciting to see it fall, but poor Mark missed it. We also had two other sections of our fence blown down by the high winds. We also lost a beautiful Christmas tree when it broke cleanly about a foot from the ground.

As the winds continued, I decided to give Mark two more vials of factor VIII early, in case the power went out. And sure enough it did! I wasn't too worried at first because I knew the pump would work on battery power for a few hours. I called the Electric Light Company. They knew we had lost our power but told us there were so many power outages that they couldn't promise we'd have electricity until the next day. So much for being on the priority list! I called the fire department and the police department to see if they could get me a generator. They said that all of theirs were being used, but they'd try to get one from somewhere. They never did. It was getting dark and Dale called her friend Mary Patricia Medeiros because she remembered that they had a generator.

Mary Patricia and I had gone to the same grammar school—Sacred Heart in Fall River—and she was a close friend of my sister. She used to live right around the corner from us. Her husband Drew went to school with Dale in Swansea. He had been in her class in grammar school. We hadn't seen each other for years until Mary Patricia entered Truesdale Hospital to have her baby. She was put in the same room with Dale and they became instant friends. Our Mark was born on August 2 and her Marc (spelled with a c) was born on August 4. The two boys remained close friends. Mary Patricia's parents and my parents were also friends.

Drew is the type of guy who would drop anything he was doing, no matter how important, to help a friend. Before long, Drew and Marc were at our house hooking up their generator for our Mark. I learned how to put the gasoline in and how it worked. We were able to keep the pump working and have a light for Mark so we could see to mix the ampicillin. I don't know what we would have done without that machine.

The next morning the power was still out and we decided that Mark would be more comfortable some place with electricity. I knew my parents had power in Fall River, so I called and asked if we could stay. I carefully carried Mark to the car and put pillows under his feet to protect his ankle. I had given him two vials of factor VIII and then had loaded all the IV equipment and medicine into the car.

Mark was still very uncomfortable with the ankle and every bump on the road hurt him. As soon as we were in Fall River, I decided to call Dr. Smith again at his home. He felt that it would be best for Mark to come back to the hospital where he could get better pain medication and they could check the ankle out again more thoroughly. So we loaded all our clothes and supplies back into the car and headed for Providence. Mark ended up in room 3 this time, right next door to his old room.

Mark seemed happy to be in the hospital again because he really felt miserable and he thought the doctors could do something to ease his pain. But he was also depressed and asked, "Why me, Dad? Why do I have to have all this bad luck? Why does everything have to happen to me?" Ninety-nine percent of the time, Mark was very positive, but this was one of those few times when we had to have a long talk.

I told him that I couldn't answer his question, but that he was not alone in his suffering. "Thousands of children are starving to death, thousands of children are in hospitals, thousands of children are being abused, thousands of children have handicaps that are even worse than yours," I told him. But he reminded me of the thousands that were perfectly healthy. His friends and classmates were all healthy. They could do whatever they wanted. He wished that he was like them. I told him that he was "special." There had to be a reason for all of his suffering. I always told him that God would have a special place for him in heaven. We can't understand God's plans for us, but someday everything will be made known to us. "Some day," I told him, "you will have the answer to your question. For now, be thankful for the positive things. Be thankful for our family. How many of your classmates come from broken homes? How many of your classmates have the special bond that we have in our family? How many of your classmates have the support of a whole town?" I went on to tell him, "The town of Swansea is behind you. People care about you. The newspapers are full of articles about the people in Swansea supporting you. I know that this can't make your ankle pain go away, or your AIDS, or your hemophilia. But how would you like to be poor Ryan White in Kokomo, Indiana? No one there seems to care about him at all. The whole town seems to be against him."

"You're right, Dad," he said. "I should write to Ryan White and tell him that I know how he feels. I can be a friend to him."

And later in the week when Mark was feeling better, we found out Ryan's telephone number and called his home. Ryan was also sick and in the hospital. His stepfather gave us the telephone number of his hospital room. Dale called Jeanne White and they had a long conversation comparing the two boys and their similar problems. Dale told her that Mark even resembled Ryan. Later Mark got to talk to Ryan and they had a good conversation about hobbies. Ryan collected comic books and G.I. Joe figures. Mark told Ryan about all his collections. He also had G.I. Joe figures. They talked about the hospital and the hospital food. Ryan told Mark that he didn't care for it and wasn't eating that well. Mark told Ryan that he had to eat to keep healthy. They promised each other that they would keep in touch through letters and an occasional phone call.

In their letters they exchanged pictures and discussed everyday things that teenagers talk about. Dale and Jeanne White continued to call each other from time to time to see how things were going. It was from Jeanne White that we found out that Ryan was on gamma globulin, a blood product that was supposed to help the immune system. We talked to Dr. Smith about it and he started Mark on it also. In fact, it was started during that hospital stay and continued at home every two to four weeks for the rest of the year.

Dr. Lucas examined Mark and decided to operate again. The operation would be a carbon copy of the last one. They would go into the ankle joint with the arthroscope to see what was going on inside. The operation was scheduled for Monday, September 30. I didn't need to take the day off from school because it was cancelled due to downed wires from the hurricane.

Once again we would walk down the long corridors with

Mark as he was pushed to the operating room. This would be his third operation since coming down with AIDS and I ached for him. It wasn't any easier for Dale and me, either, even though we had been through it before. A sense of great sadness went through me as I kissed him good-bye and wished him luck. It is impossible to describe what it feels like to experience at one and the same moment grief, anger, and the wish that it was you and not your child who had to endure such awful pain.

Mark came out of the operation fine. I prayed that the new month starting the next day would bring better luck for us all. Scott had also had a bad month. In September he had to receive 13 treatments of factor VIII—all for his left knee that was still giving him trouble. Meanwhile, he still managed to go to school each day and keep up with his work, despite being shipped around from grandmother to grandmother, never having two parents home at the same time, and visiting the hospital nightly. I asked him if anyone in school ever mentioned anything about Mark, but no one had except the teachers who always asked how Mark was doing.

Mark's ankle was still extremely sore. He was put on chlorophenical again because the doctors felt that it had worked better than the ampicillin. Salmonella was still found in the joint. Therefore, it would be quite some time before Mark would be able to go to school or even walk again. A few days after the operation, he was feeling a little better and we would take him outside in a wheelchair. They had a playground behind the Potter Building for the children who were well enough to use it and we took him out there. The weather was still good in early October and Mark loved to be outside. It was pretty with the trees turning magnificent rainbow colors. On weekends Scott also liked to be out in the back, rather than in the stuffy, small hospital room.

Mr. Devine came up to visit Mark a couple of times. Mark was very pleased that his principal would take the time to see him and tell him all about the happenings at the school. Mr. Devine would also bring messages from some of the kids. Mark had always liked Mr. Devine and before long, he was more than a principal, he was a friend to all of us.

As had happened in his previous stays, Mark had many visitors. He loved company and he especially liked getting cards in the mail. Once again we started a new collection of greeting cards on the door. Mark had all the same nurses and they gave him excellent care. None of them on the three shifts treated him any differently because he had AIDS. His stay went very smoothly except for the pain in his ankle which never did seem to go away.

Father Jim Fitzpatrick from St. John's in Attleboro came down to visit Mark. Dale and I were a little embarrassed by some of the posters that were hanging in Mark's room. My brother Jon had bought Mark three or four posters of women in bathing suits which Mark immediately had wanted hung up. We kind of tried to hide them behind the door, but most of the young interns soon spotted them. Father Jim found them and teased Mark about them.

Father Jim had known Mark through some of the various activities at my school. He had been a chaperone on all of my class trips ever since he came to St. John the Evangelist Church as a deacon. Since my boys were hemophiliacs, and since I had been the one to give the treatments, we always took the boys with us on our eighth grade trips, along with all the necessary factor VIII, syringes, tourniquets, sodium chloride, alcohol preps, gauze pads, and bandaids. Mark loved going on all of them. For our New York State trip we would get up at 4:00 A.M. so we could be in Attleboro by 5:30. The bus would come about 5:45 and I would let the chaperones board the bus first. Later the students would line up by numbers which I gave them based on behavior throughout the year. The students with the best conduct would be first and have the choice of seats.

We would then head for New York State, making a rest stop at the last restaurant on the Mass Pike. We arrived at our first destination, Howe Caverns, around 10:30 A.M. The students would take the elevator down to the caverns 200 feet below the ground. Mark loved the caverns even though we had made the trip many times before. He especially liked the underground boat ride and the walk along the "winding way." This was a very narrow passage that kept twisting and turning for about 500 feet. After walking for one and one-half miles in the cool 52 degree temperature, the lodge at the top felt nice and warm. We would have lunch and then the students would buy souvenirs and play video games. Mark and Scott both loved this part of the trip. They were excellent players.

Next we would travel a short distance in our coach to Secret Caverns, which were famous for their 100-foot underground waterfall. This was a family run business and not as famous as Howe's, but they were very different caverns and the family was very friendly. The caverns had a natural entrance and you had to walk down many stairs to enter. They were very narrow caverns and had many low hanging stalactites. Many of the students liked these caverns even better than Howe. Mark said he liked them both.

At 2:00 P.M. we would head further west to Cooperstown, New York. We arrived about an hour later and toured the Farmers' Museum. It was like a miniature Sturbridge Village in Massachusetts and very educational. Then we would go to the Baseball Hall of Fame and Museum. As an ardent fan, Mark never tired of seeing the displays. The kids all liked this, too, especially the gift shop that had just about any item that you wanted connected with the sport. And they liked the quaint little town of Cooperstown. It was a quiet place with friendly people. We would all walk down to Doubleday Field and stop at many of the shops along Main Street. Mark especially liked the ice cream parlor.

Later we would stop at McDonald's and then make one more ice cream stop before getting back to Attleboro just after midnight. It was a tiring day, but fun-filled and Mark never wanted to miss it, though he was forced to miss twice due to his hemophilia.

I didn't make my students go there every year. Each class could decide where they wanted to go by a majority vote. But the other classes liked the trip so much, they recommended it to the seventh graders, who usually voted for it when they were in the eighth grade. Three classes did go elsewhere. My first class went to Boston and two other classes went to New York City.

Seeing Father Jim reminded Mark of the trips to New York and Rocky Point, an amusement park in Rhode Island where we would go every year to ride all day and eat clam cakes and chowder—all you could eat—and watermelon, too. They were happy memories for Mark. One year he couldn't go to New York because of an ankle bleed, and the very next year it happened again. So I decided to take him anyway and carried him on my back the whole day—through the caverns and all. Mark appreciated that. Unfortunately, the bus broke down that year due to transmission problems, and we didn't get back to Attleboro until 7:00 A.M. the next morning. We had to make 40 collect calls to notify the parents that we'd be very late and call them when we got in, which probably would be in the morning. We spent half the night in an Albany bus depot, which was an education in itself.

Many teachers from my school and people from Dale's church came to the hospital to visit. Mark was always in a good mood and often would play jokes on them or perform magical tricks. He also did this with all the nurses. Dr. Smith also had tricks played on him as did the interns. Debbie DeMaio, our social worker, was one of Mark's favorite targets. Rev. Dr. Leon Tavitian, from Dale's church, did not escape the jokes either.

Mark's ankle was still very sore the whole week after the operation. Nobody knew the pain he had! But he'd still try to move around and Dale told me he would struggle to get out of bed each night so he could make Dale's bed up for her. He also cared about us not getting our proper rest and not eating well. He would order extra food on his tray for Dale and me. He was a super, caring, loving young man. No parent could ask for more in a child. Of course, he could get into some pretty good arguments with his brother at times, but most of the time he really was very well behaved.

When Mark was in Cub Scouts, he did an assignment that I treasure because it tells so much about him. In it he mentioned that his nicknames were: "Marko Polo, Marko, Marko Poloco, and Markey." He said if he could be called by another name, he'd choose "Rocky because he is a boxer." He had to list his favorite things to touch. At age 10 they were: "Wood, nails, ropes, cars, big trucks, candy, toys, campers, fur, cats, dogs, coats, ponies, baseballs, footballs, soccer balls, racquetballs, dirtbikes, sand, water, and clay." When asked to list the things he didn't like to touch, he responded: "Mud, crabs, poison, fish, ants, bugs, deadstuff, cat claws, needles, fire, top of dog food cans (he had cut himself trying to open up a can of dog food and required stitches), rocks I have stepped on with bare feet, bees, and a rock that hit me in the head." When asked if the pain was useful he put down, "Only the needles because I need my treatment to stay healthy." When asked to list his favorite smells, they were: "Roses, good cooking, being clean, smells of food, and after shave lotion." His least favorite smells were: "Smoke, cigarette smoke, skunk, rotten eggs, junk-garbage, and junk yards." He had to list his favorite things to taste. They were: "Ice cream, apples, bananas, spaghetti, pizza, fish, and clams." The tastes he didn't like were: "Sloppy Joes, iron (the liquid kind he took because of his low blood), pancakes, butter, and jelly." Some of his favorite sights were: "Sunset, trees, mountains, water, animals, and the snow." Some sights he didn't like to see were: "An animal in pain, somebody in a car accident, a fire, and two people fighting." Some of his favorite sounds were: "Birds singing, the radio, record player, music, and people clapping." Sounds he didn't like to hear were: "Loud noises, people yelling at you, scratching your fingernails against a blackboard, and a windstorm." Mark also wrote a short poem which he memorized and would always say:

My name is Mark,
I'm not afraid of the dark.
I can be a big help,
Just give me a yelp.
I try my best,
to pass the test.
Sometimes I am bad,
Sometimes I am mad,
But most of the time,
I please my mom and dad.

The Cub Scout paper asked how he felt about the dark. Mark answered: "I like it dark when I'm sleeping, and it doesn't bother me."

In a prayer he wrote to God he said: "Dear God, thank you for my brother and my father and mother. Thank you for making me born in America. Thank you for all the stuff you have done for me. But I still have one question, why did you give me hemophilia? Love, Mark Hoyle"

He had to write about a family member and chose Scott. "My best friend is Scott. Scott is my brother. Although I have many friends in school, at Cub Scouts, and in Little League. Scott is always around when I need him. We play catch together, Atari games, and ride bikes. We also know how it is to be hurt and to get treatment. That's because we both have hemophilia."

He also had to write about a friend. He chose Angel Negron. "Angel is my buddy. We ride the bus together to school. We play in the school yard. We never fight. He is a good friend to have. We buy each other presents on birthdays. I wish he lived closer to me."

Angel was a good friend of Mark's. They had been in the same class since kindergarten at the Mason Barney School in Swansea. And Mark was right, I don't think they ever had a fight.

Cub Scouting was fun and Mark enjoyed it. He went on a weekend retreat down in Westport, Massachusetts, and he also earned a religious award. He worked for the highest award in Cub Scouts, the Arrow of Light, and earned that, too. We were proud of his accomplishments in Cub Scouting, although he felt bad that the cars we made for the derby never did that well.

During Mark's second stay at Rhode Island Hospital he received a big boost in spirits from a special group that was formed to ease our family's ordeal and to show support. Here is the story of how this group was founded.

Susan Travers, the mother of three Swansea children, felt bad for our family although she had never met us. She had educated herself about AIDS and had not planned on attending the Swansea school meeting because she had no fear. But after hearing the issue discussed at corner stores and all over town, she decided to go. She wanted to be a positive voice and she did speak up at the meeting as I noted earlier. She gave a heartwarming speech in defense of our family which brought loud applause from the crowd.

The night of the meeting her husband Joe, also known as

"Trampis" by his friends, found out that the boy with AIDS was Dale Gardiner's son. Dale had gone to school with Joe and they had been very close friends. It was Tom Blakey, a Swansea police officer and a friend to both Dale and Joe, who told him. Tom Blakey had transported Mark to Fall River Pediatrics in his patrol car during the Blizzard of '78 when all the roads were closed and Mark had needed treatment. He had been very nice to Mark and even let him wear his police cap.

Dale used to babysit for Joe's family while she was in high school. Joe told his wife about the news. Later that night my brother Jeff called Sue to thank her for supporting his nephew Mark. Sue didn't know the relationship when she spoke at the meeting. Jeff had known the Travers family through the Swansea Soccer League and Swansea Independent Baseball League. My sister Jayne also knew them through the soccer and also the local football league. We didn't know Sue because, being hemophiliacs, Mark and Scott could not play football or soccer.

Now Sue felt even stronger about showing support. We were just an average family like the rest of the Swansea residents. What if this tragedy had happened to her? she wondered. How would she feel about this meeting and all the newspaper articles about her son? How would she handle this terrible health problem? One thing she knew, she would appreciate support.

Tragedy was nothing new to Sue. She had lost three family members in tragic accidents—all before they reached 25 years of age. "None of us knows when our number is up," she noted. "I wanted to give Mark a chance at life they didn't have."

One ironic part of all this was that two years after I had met Sue Travers, I found out that it was my brother Jon and myself who several years earlier had called the police to report the accident on Bushee Road where Sue's brother had died. Jon had been on his way to my house when he saw some taillights off the road in the woods. He then noticed a fence torn down and knew there had been an accident. He continued on to my house, about a minute's drive from the spot, so we could call the police and get an ambulance out there as quickly as possible. We then went back to the accident scene to show the police exactly where it was. We arrived minutes before the police and called out to see if anyone needed help, but there was no response.

The police found Sue's brother dead. I didn't know him, but I felt terrible. I remember that I couldn't sleep at all that night. My brother later told me he didn't get any sleep either.

Sue Travers talked to my sister at a football game the weekend after the Swansea meeting. She asked Jayne what she could do to help. What would we accept, what wouldn't we accept? She wanted to do something, but didn't know what. Jayne suggested talking to my brother Jeff; maybe he had some ideas of what we needed. She saw Jeff the next day at a soccer game and asked him the same question, "What can we do to help?" Should they start a petition drive in favor of Mark's attendance in school to counter the Fagundes' petition? How about mowing the lawn? They knew that Dale and I were spending every available minute at the hospital and that things weren't getting done around the house. How about raising some gas money? They knew we were doing quite a bit of traveling back and forth to the hospital. Jeff told Sue he would have to check with me first before they did anything. So Sue would come up with ideas, call Jeff, and he would call me, present the ideas, and then get back to Sue. Sue didn't know us but she continued to make more and more plans to help.

She enlisted the help of her friend Linda Nahas and her sister-in-law Robin Sherman. Linda has three children and Robin two. "What if it had been my kid?" they all wondered. "I can't imagine having to face what they're facing—alone," said Linda. Their primary objective was to "give love, support, a shoulder to cry on" to the AIDS victim and his family. They also wanted to help other parents understand that Mark was a child just like their own. "We've taken our experience as mothers and said we wouldn't want our child to be treated like this," said Sue.

The three women had no history of community activism. Sue, 32 at the time, was a telephone operator. Linda, 36, and Robin, 32, ran a housekeeping business. And they were all terrific cooks! No doubt that's why they came up with the idea of making meals for our family. They knew that we weren't eating properly at the hospital—Jeff had confirmed that—so they each called some friends and asked about cooking a meal for the family of the Swansea AIDS victim. No one they called refused. They quickly had 40 volunteers and started leaving a meal a night at my brother's house across the street. Since one of us always stayed over at the hospital with Mark, the other would come home with Scott and have a deliciously prepared meal that could be warmed in the oven or the microwave. Jeff would bring it over to us. They were indeed full course meals complete with all the trimmings, including breads, desserts, soda, and an occasional bottle of wine. Of course, there usually would be plenty left over to take up to Mark the next day to heat up in the microwave at the hospital. Mark was sick and tired of the hospital food (except for the Italian Day) and looked forward to the food from Swansea. It was an outpouring of love by these terrific, caring mothers. The meals even continued for a while after Mark got home from the hospital, but I finally had to put a stop to it because now that we were settled at home again we could do for ourselves. But they insisted on making at least one meal a week for the next several weeks because some of the mothers hadn't had a turn yet and wanted to cook for us.

But the three mothers didn't stop with meals. They found out that Mark collected autographs so they made phone calls to the Boston Celtics, Boston Red Sox, New England Patriots, etc., asking for autographs. They all responded. They also sent other items like banners, stickers, and shirts.

Linda came up with the idea of her daughter's dancing school putting on a performance to benefit Mark. They also came up with the idea of a raffle and a teenage dance. Sue would do the telephoning and Robin and Linda would go around to businesses looking for donations.

The idea of a fundraiser was to show the positive side of Mark's battle—to counterbalance Mrs. Fagundes. They talked to us first and then went to Mr. Devine. They wanted to show community support for Mark. Mr. Devine agreed to allow the students at Case Junior High to sell raffle tickets—of course, only those who wanted to sell them. Sue believes that just about all the students got involved. The secretaries at the school helped count and sort the tickets. Over $3,000 worth of raffle tickets were sold by the students alone.

The three mothers wanted a name for their group of 40 mothers and students. They didn't want any gruesome name about an AIDS victim, they wanted something positive. They came up with an idea, but first had to check with us since Mark's name had never been used by the press. We thought it was a wonderful name and from then on they were known as the "Friends of Mark."

They needed prizes for the raffle. The first place they went to was Ann & Hope, a discount department store in Seekonk, Massachusetts. They were hoping that the manager would give them a good discount on a bike, or even sell them a bike at cost. They explained why they wanted a bike at discount, and the manager said he would give them a bike for free. So the first prize was a girl's 10-speed bicycle.

They opened a post office box under the name "Friends of Mark." Sue, being an operator, thought it ironic that the number given to them was 411. The post office box served several purposes. People with questions could contact the group, donations could be made, and cards and letters could be sent to Mark without giving his address.

During the first week in October, Sue decided that she would like to visit and meet Mark. She went up to Rhode Island Hospital and met Mark and me. Dale was home at the time. She told him about all the wonderful plans they had. Mark was very excited and very thankful for everything the group was doing for him and his family. Sue felt sorry for Mark because she could see how painful his ankle was. You couldn't even sit on the edge of his bed without causing the mattress to go down and Mark to yell out in pain. Sue promised to visit him again soon.

One week later, October 8, Mark was in surgery again. This was the third operation on his ankle and his fourth operation since the onset of AIDS. The doctors were not sure he'd ever be able to walk on it again. It was very frustrating for Mark and everyone who cared about him. I took two days out of school to comfort him and Dale.

Mark continued to receive many cards at the hospital and letters from different students. Jennifer Nahas, the daughter of Linda and a seventh grade student at the junior high, wrote to tell how all the students were behind him and hoped he got well soon. She also told him that her dancing school was going to perform at the junior high for his benefit.

This event was the first in a series of ideas that had been

planned by the Friends of Mark. Pupils of Pat Medeiros' Creative Dance and Performing Arts Center of Tiverton, Rhode Island, gave a performance at Case Junior High following the school's open house for parents. Both parents and teachers enjoyed an informal coffee hour in the cafeteria and the performance in the media center. Donations were given at the performance to be added to the Friends of Mark fund, which really started to grow. The open house was held October 23. A picture of part of the dance troupe appeared in *The Spectator* under the heading: "Dancing for Mark."

Donations started coming to the post office box. Hasbro-Bradley Toys of Pawtucket, Rhode Island, not only donated items for the raffle, but also toys for both Mark and Scott.

Sue Travers told me how cooperative everyone was. "Everything just fell into place as if it was God's will that it happened," said Sue. "There were no obstacles." When asked by a reporter what the most difficult thing was that they had to face, she answered, "Nothing." It was actually fun for the three women because people cared. She received many, many positive calls.

P.D.Q. Printing and R.E. Smith Printing donated the raffle tickets. Lincoln Press donated the dance tickets and Eastern Printing donated the thank you notes which said, "Thank you! For your donation to 'Friends of Mark.' We are grateful for both your financial help and your emotional support. Mothers Chapter of 'Friends of Mark.'"

All the Parent-Teacher Organizations in Swansea sent donations as did all the fire stations, the Swansea Little League, the Swansea Independent Baseball League, and Swansea Youth Soccer League. Local variety stores, oil companies, florists, pharmacies, lumber companies, tire companies, bicycle shops, gas stations, hairdressers, restaurants, metal shops, video stores, banks, American Legion, VFW, supermarkets, and many other businesses and organizations too numerous to mention all made donations. The women kept excellent records and gave me a copy so my family would know from where all the support was coming. Many individuals also sent in donations to the post office box, including many from other states and one addressed simply to Mark, Swansea, Ma.

It was practically a full-time job contacting people, visiting the post office box, and sending thank you notes. Sue, Linda, and Robin did all this for a boy they had not even known before that year.

They sent out a news release to the press which said: "Friends of Mark, a non-profit, volunteer organization consisting of students, parents, and friends of the young Swansea AIDS victim, will sponsor two fund raising events.

"A dance for junior high school students will be held at the Bluffs Community Center in Ocean Grove in Swansea, November 2 from 7 to 10 P.M. Music will be provided by the rock group 'Tora.' Admission is $3 and all proceeds will be used to help the family defray expenses.

"The organization will also sponsor a raffle. Prizes, donated by area businesses and Swansea School PTO's include a boy's 'Predator' bike, a girl's ten speed, Trivial Pursuit, a 'boom box' radio, a skate board, a Cabbage Patch doll and a Cabbage Patch pillow."

Three newspapers printed the release. One had the heading: "Friends to help AIDS victim." Another headline was: "Friends of Mark plan fund raisers." A third had: "2 fundraisers scheduled for medical bills of boy with AIDS in Swansea."

The *Providence Journal* called Sue about the release and added a little story along with it. Sue told them how Dale had been forced to quit her job to spend more time with her "ailing son," and how I had been forced to leave a second job. She told them about Mark being in Rhode Island Hospital because of complications related to his hemophilia and how his younger brother also had hemophilia. They wrote a nice article about the community offering "time, money, and support" to our family.

Edward J. Durand, the news editor of the *Fall River Herald-News,* had a nice piece entitled: "One night the Town of Swansea turned the lights on across America." He praised the people of Swansea and, in particular, Superintendent McCarthy. "The people of Swansea—from the kids in the school system, to the woman professional and the guy working on cars out on the state highway—are standing head and shoulders above people in places like New York City and Kokomo, Ind."

Mr. Durand went on to say that Swansea was a "special place with special people. What has happened in this community has far reaching significance," he said. "It offers hope that the cloak of darkness—that has been hanging over our nation—may be driven from the land through enlightened and rational procedures and in a spirit of justice that is the life sustenance of America."

The *New Bedford Standard Times* had an editorial in which the writer criticized his own school committee in New Bedford because it wanted to isolate students with AIDS. The editor told the people to look at Swansea where an elementary school student with AIDS was admitted to school and where the community has rallied around the victim and his family. "While neighbors and friends of the family prepare meals and help in any way they can, the schoolchildren are pitching in with fund-raising to help defray the medical bills the family is faced with." State Health Commissioner Bailus Walker called Swansea a "model for the nation."

6

*"So often, our choice is between fear and
compassion. I know which one is the harder
choice. I know that across the country,
Swansea alone has made it . . . .
I thought how proud I'd be to live here."*

—Mark Patinkin in the
Providence Journal-Bulletin

Mark seemed to be doing a little better after this last operation. His ankle was still extremely sore, but his whole
attitude about it seemed more positive. He was receiving gamma
globulin for his immune system and this pleased all of us.

My parents brought some Halloween items to the hospital.
We hung the decorations on the wall in Mark's room. They also
brought a large hat and matching bow tie. Mark wanted to wear
them as a joke. He loved to clown around with everybody. Some
people from Dale's church came for a visit and we all went
down to the cafeteria to have ice cream. Mark was in a wheelchair and wore the hat and bow tie. We all had a good time that
day.

On Monday, October 14, Mark came home from the hospital. His ankle, though still painful, was improving. It was a
Monday holiday, Columbus Day, and I was able to find a parking spot right in front of the hospital. We had to make quite
a few trips to the car with the great accumulation of articles
that Mark had collected. I wondered if there would be room for
everything, but there was.

Mark was thrilled to be in the car again. The autumn foliage
was just starting to peak and Mark enjoyed the ride down I-195
to Swansea. We rented a wheelchair at Pleasant Drug in Fall
River, a store we were very familiar with since we purchased
most of our hemophilia supplies from there. It would be easier

for Mark to get around in the house and outside on the decks. We could also use it to take Mark shopping and he was at the age where he loved new clothes. On one shopping trip he picked out jogging outfits and "cool" shirts. And, of course, he had to have mousse for his hair. He also wanted a blue jean jacket. We bought him two.

Once Mark came home, the Swansea school department arranged for a tutor. Mark had kept up with his school work while at Rhode Island Hospital through a teacher who worked there. She had come to his room just about every day and later, when he was able, he had gone down to her classroom with the other ill students. Mark was always concerned with his work and had to work very hard to get the grades he received.

The Swansea tutor was Libby Hood and she taught at the junior high school. Mark really didn't like to be tutored, but he enjoyed Mrs. Hood. She would gather all the work from his teachers and leave him long assignments when she was finished. She worked with Mark for quite some time before some personal concerns forced her to quit. Kathy Ryan came in her place. It turned out that she lived on the next street over and Mark knew her daughter. Dale had known her in high school. She was also very nice to Mark.

Sue Gemma, the therapist, continued working with Mark at our home. She would come twice a week to exercise Mark. Mark would give himself treatment each time she came in order to prevent a bleed. He had light exercises to do on the days that she didn't come. He also continued to get his gamma globulin treatments at home. Nancy Keyes would come and also a nurse from the Home Nutritional Health Services. So between the tutor, therapist, and nurses, Mark was kept very busy. Many relatives and friends would also drop in to see him. Mr. McCarthy and Mr. Devine came to our house one day. It was the first time that Mark had met Mr. McCarthy and he was thrilled to meet the man who had done so much for him.

Maureen Bushell, the school nurse at Case Junior High, was another frequent visitor. She often went up to see Mark in the hospital, too. She always sent him cards and brought him presents. She was another Swansea resident who, though we had not known her before, became a great friend. It turned out that her husband Joe knew my father and worked for the same autoparts store, although a different branch. And I had picked orders for Joe when he owned his own store and I worked at Alden Autoparts.

Mark enjoyed getting mail from the Friends of Mark post office box and he was always excited to receive more autographs. Something else that brought a smile to Mark's face were the packages he received from Diamond Communications of South Bend, Indiana, publishers of sports books and calendars. Jill Langford, president, had found out about Mark through a mutual friend, Joyce Chatfield of Attleboro, Massachusetts. Diamond sent both Mark and Scott priceless autographed memorabilia, including a baseball from Joe DiMaggio, posters from Phil Cavarretta, and a book from Tiger broadcaster Ernie Harwell. When it became time to seek out a publisher for Mark's story, I immediately thought of Diamond. Jill and her husband Jim told me to look no further for a publisher. In their commitment to Mark's story, they made this book the first title of a newly-created imprint, Langford Books.

Mark never stopped talking about a dirtbike and how much he wanted to get one. Dale and I had mixed emotions about this; we knew that the whole hemophilia team in Rhode Island would be against it. Dale bought him a pair of gloves for a dirtbike and promised him she would buy him the dirtbike when he went back to school full-time.

On October 22, television crews went to Case Junior High School to interview nine students about Mark. Diane Willis of the Channel 7, WNEV News Team interviewed Heather Gregory, Kailin O'Brien, Monica Ponte, Liz Aguiar, Robyn Medeiros, Lisa Dowling, Michael Sullivan, Joey Oliveira, and Lisa Curry. Later that day they were also interviewed on the AIDS issue by Sarah Terry of WGBH-FM, Monitor Radio Network. All nine students felt that Mark belonged in school. Diane Willis devoted one whole segment of the "Young Times" news program to the interview. Here is what they had to say:

Willis: How would you feel, how would your children feel about going to school with a child with AIDS? Well, tonight on "Young Times" you will meet kids in Swansea who were the first in the country to grapple with that question. And they feel that they have made the right choice and now they want to teach us. Yesterday, for the first time, their principal allowed a reporter inside the school to get a chance to talk with them.

Gregory: I know it changed me and I mean they were waiting, I think that they were waiting for him to be here, and like with all their cameras and everything, and it was really rotten because. . . .

Willis: What angers these eighth graders the most was, as they call it, the scavenger hunt by the media to find their friend Mark. He is their classmate with AIDS. They rally around him with a fierceness of loyalty and love that makes them understand and not fear.

Ponte: He deserves exactly what we should get because he's part of this school. And if we kick him out of this school, then this school is never what it used to be. And this school is made up of education, and partly love, and we want him back.

Gregory: There's nobody here who doesn't want him back. Everybody wants him here. And like if he came back he'd just be like one of us, you know, just a normal person. It wasn't his fault that he caught it, you know, what I mean. . . .

Willis: They're just 13 and along with math and science and English, they've had to learn first hand about AIDS, and about AIDS' other name, "Fear" . . . Pretend that I have AIDS. Would you shake hands with me?

Oliveira: Sure.

Willis: Would you give me a hug?

Oliveira: Sure.

Willis: Would you give me a kiss?

Oliveira: Probably.

Willis: But certainly, this is making them feel older.

Curry: A problem with like what kind of ice cream am I gonna have, like a real serious problem that we have to think about and make a decision, and I think we made the right one.

Willis: They don't know why their school is becoming a model of tolerance around the country for a child with AIDS. But in their directness and in their honesty it all seems simple. They hope they can leave behind a lesson of love and understanding for adults.

Medeiros: At least let the people who have it, let them finish their lives that they have to live and let it be a good one.

Ponte: I know I'd want to come back and be with my friends, and just live life and just keep going until it is over.

Oliveira: He was my friend and he will be my friend until he dies.

Willis: They are so mature and they are so honest and they are so wise. They told me that Mark is doing better, he's improving and that he hopes to be back at school soon. And they say that the biggest thing they can give him is to make him forget that he has AIDS and to feel just as he did last year.

Mrs. Hood told Mark that he needed to do an autobiography for his English class. I'd like to share this assignment with you:

It was a bright sunny day when I came into this world (so they tell me). August 2, 1972, was the big occasion, at 8:30 A.M. My father was James and my mother Dale, and I was their first born. I had my parents all to myself until March of 1975 when my brother Scott was born. My mother was home all day and worked a few nights a week at Sears. My father taught school in Attleboro. As a family we were always very close and still are to this day. We live at 51 Lockewood Circle in a nice green house with a stockade fence around the whole backyard. The backyard is my favorite place because we have a screened-in patio, two decks, a swimming pool and two tree houses.

My biggest hobby is collecting baseball cards. I have been doing it since I was a kid, but the past couple of years I have really gotten into it. I have a Red Sox collection that is my specialty (over 1100 cards), but I also collect complete sets. I have 18 complete sets. My other hobby is collecting autographed pictures and other items. I have a hockey stick signed by the Bruins, Kelly Tripucka's own basketball shirt, Russ Gibson's baseball, autographed baseball cards of the whole team of the Waterbury Indians, and many other items.

Baseball has always been my main interest. I have been in the Swansea Little League since I was 8. I played for championship teams and losers, but it was always fun. I played shortstop and pitched. Another interest is my animals. We have four cats, a dog, a parakeet, and tropical fish. "Champ" is my favorite cat. Wrestling and the Red Sox are my two favorite TV programs. Although I have a lot of other favorite shows, too. Eating shrimp at a restaurant is another thing I like to do. Bowling, golf, and the show are some of my other favorites. I took golf lessons this summer and enjoyed it very much.

When I grow up, I'd like to own a baseball card shop. A 4x4 vehicle is what I want to drive.

Walt Disney World was probably the most exciting thing I did in my life. I enjoyed everything about Florida and would love to go back again some day. Every vacation has been exciting. I have visited many states.

My main concern is my health. Other concerns are school and my pets.

Mark got an A for this assignment and a comment from the teacher, "Very nice job, Mark."

Another exciting night for Mark was the time that Rosemary Baker came to our house. She was the friendly lady who was in charge of the local organization called "A Wish Come True." She came to visit with Mark and to offer him any wish that he wanted. Their organization earned money through various fundraisers and then it spent it on terminally ill children. Doctors would recommend children to her who qualified. The children could wish for anything that their hearts desired and the group would try its best to make their dream come true. Most of the children had picked Florida vacations to Walt Disney World. But others had picked trips to other parts of the United States and some just wanted simple requests like meeting a movie star or getting a dog.

Rosemary said that Mark didn't have to decide that night. She wanted to give him some time to think, and she would call back next week.

Dale and I told Mark that the decision would be completely up to him and we would back him 100%. We personally thought he would pick a trip since he loved vacations, but he didn't. I think his ankle was just too sore and it wouldn't have been too much fun walking on crutches.

Instead he wished for a video game. Not just one of the TV kind like "Atari," which he already had, but a regular full-size video game that you find at the malls. His favorite was a new game just out called "Paperboy." It had a handle like the front of a bike and you had to drive through all these obstacles delivering your newspapers. That's the one for which he asked.

Rosemary told Mark that she would do her best to get him one. There were different problems that came up and long delays, but Rosemary came through in the end and Mark received his video game.

It was delivered on a cold night that winter and set up in Mark's room. It seemed to weigh a ton. Steve Beckler of Beck's Games and Electronics of Seekonk, Massachusetts, set it all up for Mark and explained everything there was to know about it. "You'll never ever have to use coins in this machine," he said. "Just plug it in and it will come right on." And sure enough, he was right.

Mark loved his new game and spent many hours at it. He was able to sit on a bar stool and play, so it didn't bother his ankle at all. Scott also had much enjoyment from it. His brother was glad to share it with him (as long as he wasn't playing it at the time).

Meanwhile the Friends of Mark were still busy with their plans for the upcoming raffle and dance. We had met Robin and Linda for the first time when they delivered meals to our house. They continued to drop in on Mark to say hello.

October brought a new addition to our household. Scott's cat Tiger didn't come home one morning and we never saw it again. Scott was heartbroken, even though we had Champ, Spooky, and Dirty. Tiger was his personal cat. Champ was Mark's personal cat and Spooky and Dirty belonged to everyone.

Dale felt sorry for Scott because he had been shipped from relative to relative so much during Mark's hospital stays. She asked him if he wanted a new kitten and of course he did. Off they went to the Animal Rescue League in Fall River. Mike Alphonso, a kind, pleasant man, who had run the league for years and was a good friend of my father, saw to it that Scott had a nice choice. Scott picked a light tan and white kitten and named it Frisky for obvious reasons. Now we had four cats in the house again.

Mark loved all the cats and begged us for another new kitten for himself. We really didn't want to get another one, but then our dog Cleo, who we had for 15 years, took sick and had to be put to sleep. So to ease the pain of Cleo's departure, we decided Mark could get a new kitten, too. By chance, Dale's Uncle Nebe called to see if we wanted a kitten. A cat had a new litter in a barn near his house. We went up to see them and they were all adorable. Mark fell in love with a tiny, furry one. All our other cats were males and had short hair. This cat was also a male, but had long hair. It looked almost like an angora.

Mark took the kitten home and named it Tiny. The name fit him well at first, but before long he was bigger than all the other cats we had. He was a very loveable kitten like Champ, and they both loved to sit on Mark's lap. They would even stay there when Dale gave Mark rides in the wheelchair around the backyard.

Mark Patinkin, of the *Providence Journal-Bulletin*, talked to Sue Travers about doing an interview with Mark. She told him that she would talk to us and get back to him. She called my brother Jeff first and found out that we liked Mark Patinkin's column. However, if we were to do an interview, it would be a one-shot deal only. We didn't want to open up a can of worms and have every newspaper in the area calling for interviews. We also didn't want our last name made public. Mark Patinkin agreed to this, he just wanted to show that our Mark was a normal 13-year-old boy.

Sue Travers made all the arrangements and a date was set when I would be home from school. We were very nervous about it because we had never been interviewed by a newspaper reporter before. Mark came and I escorted him into the family room where Mark was waiting. Mr. Patinkin was dressed in a business suit and looked a great deal younger than we had expected. He had a small notebook and pen and jotted some things down as he made small talk with us. Later, we took him down to Mark's bedroom to see his card collection and autographs. We enjoyed talking with him and Mark was thrilled to meet a celebrity columnist. "They haven't beaten AIDS in Swansea, but they've stymied fear" was the headline. Here is the piece he wrote, reprinted here with his permission:

My first thought was that the neighborhood looked like the backdrop to "Leave It To Beaver." The houses were modern. Children went by on bikes. The lawns were perfect. I knocked on the door.

Mark was waiting in the next room. The only sign of the illness was that he seemed a bit thin. He is 13 now. It is hard enough to be that age when things are routine. I wondered how you begin to cope when you happen to have AIDS.

I'd agreed not to use his full name. His parents are trying hard to keep things normal. Still, they felt it was time to talk. Their community, Swansea, has been the only one in the country to let a child with this disease attend school. The father felt it only right to let his neighbors glimpse his boy.

I noticed that one wall was lined with Little League trophies. I asked what position he plays. You tend to do that in such a situation—look for reasons to avoid the subject.

"Short," he said. "And pitcher."

He has dark hair and dark eyes. (Actually Mark's eyes are hazel.) He's one of these 13-year-olds who talks faster than that guy in the old Federal Express commercial. His father mentioned he collects autographs.

"Which ones?" I asked.

"I've got Larry Bird," said Mark. "I've got Johnny Bench. Gary Carter. People like that."

"Who's Gary Carter?" said his mother.

Mark looked like it was the dumbest question he'd ever heard.

"A baseball player," he explained.

By now, the subject was hanging over us. I asked if he was having any problems with it these days. I was careful to use the word "it."

"With AIDS?" said Mark. "No. Not really."

"He had the double pneumonia in June," his father said, "but he got over that. He even went back to Little League."

Mark mentioned that he wrote Ryan White, the boy in Kokomo, Ind., who has been barred from school.

"I wanted to tell him he's not the only one who has to face all this," he said. The two also talked briefly by phone. They told each other to keep eating—for strength.

"I guess that's what mothers are for," I said. "To remind you."

His mother smiled. "To be a nag," she said.

"She doesn't really nag," I said. "Does she?"

Mark paused, then spoke. "Sometimes," he said.

We began talking about his other interests. He collects baseball cards and likes TV wrestling, especially something called the suplex.

"That's where one guy picks up the other guy and drops him backward," said Mark.

"Wonderful," said his mother.

I'd been saving a question. I knew it could be a sensitive area, so I didn't want to touch it at first. Now it seemed time.

I asked if there had been much hate mail. Or difficult phone calls.

They said there had not been a single case.

"How about friends keeping their distance?" I asked.

Again, no.

"They know Mark's pretty responsible," his father said. "He's been giving himself his factor VIII for at least three years. For his hemophilia. He's careful."

Before I sat down with them, I thought this would end up being a story of hidden controversy. It is an issue of emotion. In New York, 10,000 parents boycotted against an AIDS child.

I expected to find some of that anger here, at least beneath the surface. But it hasn't happened. There has been only support. Every night, for weeks, neighbors have been bringing over meals—anything to make things easier.

The parents attribute most of it to their school's officials. They made sure the debate was over truth, not paranoia. That is the key, the parents explained—understanding.

We stopped by his room on my way out. It is as good a glimpse into the world of a 13-year-old boy as I can imagine. There are posters of Rambo and Hulk Hogan on the door. He used to have posters of women on the walls, but he took them down to make room for sports figures. There are clear priorities here.

I stood to leave. I shook his hand. I asked if he had any advice for other children who are ill.

"Just think about good things," he said. "Over and over. I'm going to beat it. I'm going to beat it. That's what I try to do."

There is a new group in Swansea called Friends of Mark. They will be holding a dance and raffle to raise money. It is run by a woman named Susan Travers. I called her, presuming she was a family friend. In fact, she'd never met Mark's family.

"So why start this group?" I asked.

Her answer was simple.

"I have kids of my own," she said.

It struck me that the parents who marched against AIDS children elsewhere did so for the darker side of that very reason.

So often, our choice is between fear and compassion. I know which one is the harder choice. I know that across the country, Swansea alone has made it. And as I drove out of the perfect American neighborhood, I thought how proud I'd be to live here.

Halloween came and Mark asked if he could pass out the candy at the front door. He sat on a bar stool right at the door so he did not have to put any pressure on his ankle. We had over 150 children come to our door, this was about average for Halloween. Scott dressed up as Pee Wee Herman.

During the evening, Linda Nahas came over with her children—Jennifer, Ryan, and Jason. Her sister, Sharon Marchand, who was a member of the Friends of Mark and lived in Somerset, Massachusetts, also came with her daughter Becky. Sharon had cooked us some tasty meals and it was nice to meet her. Becky was dressed as Pee Wee Herman, too. Scott and Becky, both the same age, hit it off well together and started exchanging letters. Ryan, who was dressed as a girl, was the same age as Scott, too, and became a good pal. His costume was very original and I really believed he was a girl. When Scott went to Case Junior High in 1986, Ryan ended up in his class.

Jennifer Nahas had written to Mark in the hospital and he was happy to meet her. He had seen her picture in the newspaper when she danced at the junior high and thought that she was very cute. Jason was the smallest in the group, but he had a bubbly personality, so you couldn't forget that he was there.

October faded into history and I wasn't sorry to see it leave. Scott had a difficult month with his left knee and right elbow. I had to give him 15 vials of factor VIII for these problems and a bleed into his ring finger on his left hand. Dr. Smith started talking about a knee operation for Scott if things didn't improve, and we prayed that he wouldn't need it. But we had great faith in Dr. Smith, and would have listened to him if he wanted it done tomorrow.

Mark usually spent a good portion of his mornings in bed. He tried to get some exercise by walking around the yard on his crutches. He even would rake leaves while on his crutches. His ankle was still sore, but improving.

Sue Travers came to visit one morning. Mark was lying in the family room on the couch. Sue went out to see him and he said hello and then asked her what she thought dying would be like. She was kind of shocked with the question, but answered him as best she could. It surprised me to learn Mark had asked her that question, too. Usually I was the only one who would get those deep questions.

The Friends of Mark wanted to solicit donations at the Swansea Mall but they were told by Debbie Demeo, spokesperson for the mall and not to be mixed up with Debbie DeMaio the social worker, that this was against the mall policy. Later, she called Sue back to tell her they could have a booth at an upcoming special show if they sold something. The three mothers got together and decided to sell balloons. Some helium in a large tank and a small tank was donated, as were colored ribbons to tie the balloons and a wishing well to put money in. The balloons were purchased at a special wholesale price.

The mall gave the Friends of Mark an excellent spot right in the center of things and articles about the "Swansea case" were displayed so people could see what this was all about. Two signs were posted. One said, "All proceeds to benefit Mark. Won't you help?" The other said, "Please help. Thank you. Swansea Youth Stricken with AIDS. Thank you. Thank you. Thank you. Thank you." Sue, Robin, Linda, Sharon, and my sister-in-law Anne all sold balloons. Many kids from the junior high also volunteered their time. They started selling balloons Friday morning, November 1, when the mall opened, and continued the whole day. The next day they were there all day until it was time to go to Mark's dance. On Sunday, they were all back there again. The balloon sales were so successful more helium had to be purchased. The husbands helped out with this task, since the tanks were so heavy. Many people just made donations and did not take the balloons.

Dennis B———, one of the parents who had spoken against Mark's being allowed in school, bought a balloon and said he hoped that Mark would recover soon from his ankle problems and be able to go to school again. He had changed his views. Sue told reporters, "To me, this was a tremendous vote of confidence because he turned the other way. That's what we want to see, the positive taking over where the negative had been."

Sue's husband Joe was her answering service at home. Phone calls were coming in from *Newsweek, TIME, People,* and all the national news stations. Meanwhile local camera crews were at the mall interviewing Sue.

Dyana Koelsch of "Newswatch 10" in Providence was at the mall and the camera showed a large group of people purchasing balloons. Sue told her, "Mark is home, he's not active in his AIDS right now, he's doing well, his spirits are tremendous. I think he's very hopeful as we all are." Koelsch told how many parents were concerned when the news was first announced. The film showed the Swansea meeting. But now parents were trying to show some support for Mark as well as the students who had always supported him. Sue continued to say, "We have grandmothers who have called that want to help, who don't have any kids in the junior high school. We have the town nurses who have called in support. We have other parents at the high school that have called. . . ." The reporter told about Mark's ankle problem and then said, "The Swansea Mall has agreed to help. It'll take all the money that is thrown into this fountain here and give it to Mark to help out."

Saturday, November 2, was the day of Mark's dance. The Bluffs Community Center in Ocean Grove, Swansea, would be the site. While the wives were busy selling balloons, the husbands were cleaning the hall and putting up decorations.

The Coca-Cola Company donated all the soda and cups. Ocean Grove Bakery, Bess Eaton Donuts, Old Time Donuts, and Dunkin Donuts all sent pastry. The Friends of Mark mothers, the same women who had cooked for us, made goodies too, which were sold at the dance.

Mr. Devine had given Sue the name of a band which had volunteered to play for Mark. Even though the group, Tora, had another engagement scheduled, they cancelled it so they could play for free for Mark's benefit. They only had two weeks' notice, but they really came through.

Many magazines and TV stations called Sue wanting to cover the dance. She told them that the dance was really for the kids and that the press wasn't invited. As it was, Channel 12 of Providence did send Chris Luke and a camera. They had not called beforehand and weren't aware that the press would not be allowed. But since they had come all the way from Providence, Sue decided to let them in. She also admitted some newspaper reporters who showed up at the door.

More than 300 people went to the dance for Mark, including most of my eighth grade class from Attleboro and a good number of seventh graders, too. Of course the large majority of the kids came from Case Junior. Many sixth grade mothers let their daughters go because it was such a good cause. Yellow, orange, and blue balloons dangled from the ceiling. A large banner reading "We Miss You Mark" hung on a wall. The music was loud and wonderful as Tora belted out Van Halen tunes.

Chris Luke told her audience how this was "more than a Saturday night teen dance." The youngsters were there to raise funds for their classmate Mark. She interviewed my nephew Matthew Wilson, my sister's oldest child, who told her that Mark was in good spirits. "Before he couldn't really walk on his leg and now he's starting to put it down and everything. And he told me he was going to go to the dance, but I don't know."

We had a good laugh over this last comment by Matt. Here we are trying to keep the press away and he's telling her Mark is coming. Later she interviewed Joey Travers, Sue's son, who said, "The doctors said if people gave him all the spirit he could get, he would start gradually getting better and he is gradually getting better. He's looking great!"

Chris Luke noted that: "Tonight's festive atmosphere is quite different from the anxiety that prevailed in this community this past September, when it was learned that young Mark had been diagnosed with the deadly disease and wanted to return to school." The film showed pictures from that meeting and she told how Swansea was the only community to rally behind an AIDS victim.

Mark wanted to go to the dance, but he was a little bit afraid. He hadn't been in school since early September when most of his classmates hadn't known about the AIDS. He wondered how they would react to him, what they would say.

We didn't want Mark's picture plastered all over the newspapers so Scott and I went down to the Bluffs to check out the situation. Chris Luke was still there. Everyone seemed like they were having a real great time. My students came over to me and asked where Mark was. I told them that he was home, but would probably be coming later. I talked to my brother Jeff and various people on the committee and then we left.

Mark was all spruced up and ready to go when I returned. I drove back to the dance and Dale and Mark remained in the car while I went in to make sure all the press had left. All the newspaper reporters had left, but the TV people were still there. I went back to tell Mark that he would have to wait a little longer before he could go in.

It felt funny to be hiding like this, but we thought it was best. From our car we watched the TV crew leave and put their equipment in their automobile. As they pulled out of the parking lot, we got out of the car and went in.

Mark was on crutches with his foot in a cast. He walked in and at first nobody noticed him. Most of the crowd was up dancing or sitting near the band. Mark wondered where he should go and felt a little awkward. I told him that he should just sit down at one of the tables in the middle of the hall until his friends spotted him. He asked me to go with him for moral support. I helped move some chairs out of the way and he made his way to a table. Some of his friends noticed him and they came running to join him at the long, narrow table. I just left Mark there with his friends and before long others were standing around Mark asking him how he was doing. I guess the word spread that Mark had arrived because all of a sudden the whole crowd just charged to his table to be around Mark. Many stood on the other tables to get a glimpse of him. It was a heart-warming scene and it was a moment I'll always cherish. I felt so happy for the support that these kids gave him. I felt so terrific for Mark. Everyone welcomed him and shook his hand and the band, now aware that Mark had arrived, also welcomed him over the mike. It was like a scene from a movie that brought tears to your eyes.

Mr. Devine and the other chaperones had to go in and tell the kids to get off the tables before they collapsed and someone got hurt. Everyone was very cooperative. Mark had a ball. Of course, he didn't dance. He couldn't because of his ankle, but many of the girls had asked him to dance, which thrilled him. The year before he had gone to his first dance on October 26 at the junior high school. His good friend Joey Oliveira went with him and then Joey slept over at our house afterwards. Both boys were too bashful to dance that night.

We decided to leave before the last dance because we wanted to avoid the rush at the door. We slowly made our way to the car and drove back to our home. Mark was in a great mood.

The local papers covered the event. "Swansea rallies behind Mark" read the headline above a front page *Providence Journal* picture that showed a bunch of kids enjoying the dance. The *Journal* also had the headline: "Legion of friends lifts AIDS victim's spirits"—and indeed they had.

Mark had told Sue Travers how lucky he was to be accepted by his friends. "This is the only place in the country where this is happening, isn't it, Mrs. Travers?" Mark had asked as we left the hall.

"I think you can be afraid of the disease itself," said Sue to a reporter, "but you have to have compassion for the family and what they are going through."

Jessica Pineault, a Case Junior High School seventh grader at the dance, said, "We all think Mark's cool. He was very popular, still is and always will be." Serena Avant said that they all had come because of Mark. "He's an awesome kid. I've known him since the third grade."

"We Love Children," a local group from Fall River, presented Sue with a check for $250 from their organization. Many others who donated money to the Friends of Mark were complete strangers. A $100 check came from a person in Johnston, Rhode Island, for example.

The band Tora said they never thought twice about performing a free concert for Mark. The band members are Mike Morky, Vic Pontes, Lisa Furtado, Mark Furtado, and Augie Pimental. The bass player said that they were all aware of the AIDS hysteria, but realized there was an innocent teenager involved. "If I was dying from something like that I'd hope someone would help me."

Sue Travers was especially thrilled with the turnout. "This gives him a great deal of hope," she said. "He has a lot of reasons to want to get well. What we are telling him is don't you give up because we are not giving up.

"This dance made history. It was the first community sponsored dance for an AIDS victim in the country. People in New York are holding protest marches. But here in Swansea people have rallied around Mark and his parents. People have demonstrated compassion. People have confronted their fears about the unknown and looked beyond that to the boy and his family," Sue stated.

She went on to say that, "In no way do we consider his case to be terminal. We are hopeful about his future. His appetite is coming back. His doctors are very pleased with his progress. I am so proud of Swansea. A lot of people are waiting for Swansea to go up in smoke over this AIDS issue. Instead, the community has shown its support for Mark and will continue to do so."

The next day, Mark wanted to go to the Swansea Mall to watch Pat Medeiros' Creative Dance and Performing Arts students perform for him. We put the wheelchair in the trunk of the car and headed down there. We came across the Friends of Mark selling their balloons. The dancers were sitting around getting ready to perform.

They put on an excellent show and a large crowd gathered to watch them. Both our boys enjoyed the girls in their dancing costumes and wanted to stay to watch their next performance later that afternoon. Linda Nahas introduced all the girls to Mark and they all shook his hand. Later I learned how happy they were to meet the boy for whom they were dancing.

Mark enjoyed getting out of the house. It had been his first time at the mall since the summer. Of course, we didn't identify Mark to any of the people in the mall, only to the girls who had danced for him.

Sears, Roebuck and Company at the Swansea Mall sent Mark a large homemade card with $300 enclosed. Everyone signed it. It had a picture of two ballplayers talking, with the ball field in the background. "C'mon Mark, get better quick, you're up next," it said. Mark really appreciated their concern. It was the second time that he had received a large sum of money. Workers at the Catholic Memorial Home in Fall River had also chipped in for him.

My brother Jeff went to some classes at Rollins Cablevision to learn about working a video camera. At the end of the course, he could borrow one to take pictures. He asked us to come over so we could be on TV. Mark wanted to go first. He took the mike in his hand and this is what he said:

"Hello out there. This is Mark Hoyle. I'm into baseball cards. I'm going to talk about my collection. I have over 15,000 cards. My most expensive card is about $20. I have cards in drawers, in closets, under beds, and all these other odd places. I keep my cards in plastic pages to protect them. I have about 21 books full of them. I also collect complete sets, that means that there are about 600 or 700 cards published by each company that year and it comes in one big box.

"And I have an autograph wall. I have pictures of other baseball players like Johnny Bench, Gary Carter, and all the big stars. I have a hockey stick of all the Bruins—autographed, of course. And I have the Celtics starting lineup. And I have the Patriots, like Roland James and other people.

"I just got my own room and I've just redone it. Well, my baseball career started when I was only that little—(gesturing with his hand) very little, of course, and I've been collecting items up until now. I like to go to flea markets with my dad and get baseball cards.

"Every once in a while some people come over and I show them my cards. They go, 'Mark, what a wonderful collection you have, I am so impressed!' Well, I just sit back and I tell them, 'Yes, I know, I'm so great.'

"I also have pictures of Wade Boggs, Al Nipper, people like that on another wall in frames—the whole wall is filled.

"Well, that's enough about baseball, I just want to mention one more thing. I'm getting a KDX 80 dirtbike and pretty soon you'll be seeing me on it. Huh! Good-bye."

Later on Mark was interviewing me. He called it the Marvelous Mark Show and was teasing me about putting on weight, etc. I replied with the comment, "It comes with age, some day you'll be my age." Mark answered me, "I'll never be that old."

On Wednesday, November 6, we had an appointment with Dr. Smith at Rhode Island Hospital. Blood was taken and Mark's white blood count was still extremely low at 1.1 (1100) and so was his hemoglobin at 9.7. Dr. Smith thought he looked good, though, and his ankle was coming along. He suggested that Mark go back to school part-time. He arranged with Mr. Devine so that Mark could take all of his important classes in the morning, and then skip the study halls, gym classes, etc., in the afternoon. This would mean a four-hour school day with plenty of time for an afternoon nap. He would still keep the tutor for a while until we made sure that he was strong enough to handle this new situation. Walking up and down the stairs on crutches to his various classes would take a lot out of him. When he was stronger, he would be able to go the full day.

Mark was anxious to see all his friends and return to school. His friend Angel Negron had been over and he had seen some friends at a football game. But he was still apprehensive about how he would be treated, even though Joey Oliveira had talked to Mark many times on the phone and told him not to worry about anything.

It was arranged for Mark to start on Friday, the 8th. Since Monday was Veterans' Day he would have a three-day weekend to recuperate. I planned on bringing him to school in the morning so he wouldn't have to take the bus with his crutches. Dale would pick him up at noon with her mom and stepfather Tony. Later Dale's mom and Tony picked him up alone. Once in a while Uncle Leo would get him. We didn't have a second car.

The first day back, Dale borrowed her mother's car and took him in because Mr. Devine was planning to meet Mark at the door at 8:00 A.M. and that is the time I was supposed to be in Attleboro. Dale was worried that he would fall down the stairs. We had bought Mark a backpack for his books so that his hands would be free to hold the crutches.

How would you feel if you were Mark? You're at the age when everything you do: how you dress, how you act, how you talk, must meet with the approval of your peers. At that age you're more interested in feeling like part of the group than anything else. You don't want to make any mistakes in front of your classmates and look like a fool. You don't want to feel embarrassed—that's the worst feeling for a kid that age! It is easy to imagine Mark's worries: Would the kids stare at him? Would he be embarrassed and feel out of place? Would they treat him differently? I had mixed emotions myself. Case Junior had 653 students and 50 teachers. That's 700 possible responses.

The first day set the tone for the rest of the year. Everyone made Mark feel right at home again. Kids he didn't even know would speak to him. When he changed classes and walked down the corridors, he would get "Hi Mark, Hi Mark, Hello Mark, How's it going Mark? Hello Mark, Hi Mark!" Kids would go out of their way to hold doors for him or carry books or do anything they could to help. All of the teachers were just as friendly.

Mark was tired when Dale picked him up. But he was in a great mood and told her how supportive everybody was. She was pleased that everything went so well.

That night they had the first dance of the year at the junior high. The Friends of Mark asked me to go because they were going to draw the winners of the raffle during the dance. Mark didn't attend because he said he was too tired.

Scott and I went down and helped carry the prizes in from Joe Travers' truck. We put them on display in the cafeteria. The kids had worked very hard selling the tickets. Over $5,000 was made on the raffle. The winning tickets were pulled, prizes awarded to those in attendance, and then we loaded the other prizes back onto the truck to be delivered to the winners who were not present.

November was a busy month for Mark. Besides going to school he had nine sessions with his therapist, two with the social worker, and two with Nancy Keyes, the head nurse at the Hemophilia Center. She came to the house for his gamma globulin treatments and also to give him a flu shot and two pneumonia shots. Mark's arms swelled up from the shots and he had to get factor VIII for a couple of days. Altogether he had 11 vials of the clotting factor in November. Scott had 13 for his right elbow, left knee, and a flu shot.

Mark's biggest thrill that month, besides the dance, was going to the New England Patriots game. Ray Brennan, a former next-door neighbor for 12 years, gave us tickets on the 50-yard line, about half way up the stands. It was a beautiful fall day and the seats were excellent. It was a new experience for all of us because we had never been there before. The stadium was very impressive. The kids laughed when the crowd started chanting: "Tastes great! Less filling! Tastes great! Less filling!" The only bad part of the afternoon was that Scott got an unexpected beer bath! We left during the last quarter to avoid the rush at the end of the game. I gave Mark a piggyback ride to the car. We listened to the rest of the game on the car radio. The Patriots won over the Indianapolis Colts by a large margin.

It was conference time at Scott's school and as we made our way down the corridor to Mrs. Friar's fifth grade room, Mr. Dave Souza, Scott's teacher the year before, came out to greet us.

Mr. Souza wanted to know how we were doing and asked if we would mind if he took the two boys out to lunch some day. We told him it was fine with us and we'd check with the boys later—they were sitting out in the car. He called the next day to see if they wanted to go and they did.

Mark and Scott never really went any place without us. We didn't want them to get a bleed when we weren't around. But they wanted to go so we let them. A date was set up for the day after Thanksgiving. Everyone would be out of school that day.

Thanksgiving came and we continued to follow tradition. We had dinner at Dale's mother's with her brother and his family and then went back to my parents' house for sandwiches at night.

When I read the *Providence Journal* that Thanksgiving morning, I came across their editorial which was entitled: "On being plain neighborly with heartfelt thanks." I read about half of it when I came across a section talking about my son: "Black, white, Asian, whatever. It's made no difference. Kids are kids and they all deserve a chance. That's what the fellow beings in Swansea think neighbor Mark deserves." The piece went on to tell who Mark was and how the town had supported him and how the Friends of Mark had sponsored fundraisers to help our family. It mentioned the girl who said that Mark was "very popular, still is, and always will be." It then stated: "He is also very lucky—and always will be. Mark, at 13, has learned what some people never fully comprehend: the value of pure, unbounded love—even when bestowed by strangers. But he is, after all, a neighbor, and is thus entitled to receive kindness on this holiday and every day, with thanksgiving."

On this Thanksgiving Day we thanked God for Mark's health and prayed that he'd recover fully from the virus. We were all very confident that he would. So many people were praying for him that he just *had* to get better.

Scott entertained us at both houses by doing impressions of Pee Wee Herman and then changing his costume to do "The Boss"—Bruce Springsteen. Mark enjoyed his brother's show.

The "We Love Children" organization gave Dale membership card number three for Mark. This group was founded to help with those expenses not covered by medical insurance for families of children traumatized by accidents or sudden illnesses. It was founded in 1983 by Joseph Cassidy and his wife Irene when they recognized the needs of the Mikey Almeida family of Tiverton, Rhode Island. Mikey was the recipient of two liver transplants. Sue had been given a check at the dance for Mark. Dale and my mother went down to their fundraising kick-off at Chuck-E-Cheese.

The day after Thanksgiving was bright and sunny. Mark and Scott were looking at the clock as they waited for Mr. Souza to come. He was going to take them to Newport, Rhode Island.

They had a ball! They went to various gift shops and novelty shops, had a big meal and ice cream, and walked all over the Brick Market Place along Newport's waterfront. Mark was a little tired when he arrived home, but he looked great in his new red-hooded sweatshirt that Mr. Souza had bought for him. Scott could have had one too, but he chose a white Newport T-shirt instead. When it came time for Mark to have his picture taken for the school yearbook, he chose to wear the red sweatshirt that Mr. Souza had bought him.

Mark continued to remind us about the dirtbike he wanted so much. He also sent us notes and letters from time to time. Here is one of them:

To Mr. & Mrs. Hoyle.
Dear Dad and Mom,
The reason I am writing to you is I am wondering when you will let me buy my KDX 80? You know I am trying very, very hard to walk. So please can we get it on Monday, that is tomorrow. Pretty please? I love that bike very much. Please dad, I don't want to ride it until I am back to school full time. How about it, please? Remember, if you buy it pretty soon you will save $70 because it's on sale for $829. Plus, I don't want any other person to buy it. I love you guys very much. It would make me the happiest kid in the world you know. I just want to have it in my house, and sit on it. Please mom and dad? Please dad and mom, I really love that bike. Please let me get it tomorrow it would save you $70 plus make your son very, very, very, happy. You *know* that I am trying to walk as fast as I can. I don't want to be on these stupid crutches any longer. But my ankle is still stiff. I keep doing my tightening every hour. So please let me get that bike. That's the one I want.

Love, Mark

With Mark asking us every day and with letters like this, how could we not get it for him? The day we returned the wheelchair, Saturday, November 30, we bought the KDX 80 Kawasaki on the way home. It would be delivered the following week.

As November passed and December dawned, Mark continued to get stronger and healthier. He kept up with his school work and made the honor roll first term even though he had missed so much school. We continued to go baseball card hunting at card shows, card shops, and flea markets, and his collection grew steadily. Dr. Mucciardi had also scheduled a lung scan and a series of X-rays and they confirmed the good news that Mark's lungs were perfect!

The smile on Mark's face was never brighter than when his dirtbike arrived. He sat on it, inspected it, and just enjoyed owning it. We thought it best that he learn to ride it in the backyard. He studied the manual and then he was ready to try it.

I decided to ride behind him on the bike. I don't know how much help I would have been if something went wrong, but I was there anyway. Mark had problems starting it because he couldn't use his left ankle, nor stand on it to use the other foot. So I usually started it for him. He gave it some gas, let up on the clutch, and off we went in a large oval around the backyard. Mark was ecstatic! Soon I was standing on the side watching as Dale took pictures. Mark looked like he had driven it all his life. His green helmet and gloves matched the green dirtbike perfectly.

Although the weather was cold, Mark didn't feel the chilly winds at all. As we watched from inside the sliding doors in our kitchen, Mark rode round and round for hours. We had bought Scott a helmet, too, and Scott enjoyed sitting on the back for a ride.

Mark also rode around on the front lawn. We were so happy that we bought it for him, but we decided it would be best not to tell anyone at the Hemophilia Center.

It soon became apparent that our yard was just too small. It wasn't good for the bike either to be driven only in first or second gear. He asked his Nana Fazzina if he could keep his bike in her garage. They had big open fields next to her house and paths that led down to the woods.

If Mark could keep it there, he could really have some fun. Dale's mom said, "Of course you can, honey." We brought the bike down and Mark took it out to the fields. He made his own paths and could go a little faster and really enjoyed himself.

Marc Medeiros, who also had a dirtbike, would have his father bring his bike over too and together they would ride for hours and hours. They made paths through the fields and over hills and into the woods. Eventually Marc Medeiros just left his bike with Mark's in the garage because they rode them so often.

Devil's Rock was a few miles away; it was as high as a four- or five-story building and longer than three football fields. The boys enjoyed using the paths through the woods to get there and Mark, even with the bad foot, would climb to the top to explore the strange footprints that the Indians had said were made by the devil. Nearby was Margaret's Cave. It was named after an Indian who sheltered Roger Williams during the winter of 1635–36 on his way to founding Rhode Island.

Mark rode his dirtbike two or three times a week that winter. When Marc Medeiros couldn't come, he rode it by himself. We felt better when he was with Marc, but Mark usually stayed closer to his grandmother's when he was alone.

As the holidays approached, we wanted to send a thank you to all the people who had been so nice to our family. This is, in part, what I wrote in a letter I sent to four newspapers: "At this special time of the year, we would like to extend holiday greetings and thanks to everyone who has shown support for our family. Your prayers, cards, letters, meals, gifts, phone calls, visits, etc., have meant so much. . . .

"Mark is getting stronger each day. He has been attending school since early November and is very happy to be back with his friends again. We are proud to live in Swansea and so fortunate to have so many old and new friends.—The Family of Mark"

Everything seemed to be going so smoothly. But then I had this terrible nightmare. Mark was drowning in our bath tub! I saw him with frightening clarity. He was just staring up at me. It really scared me and woke me up. I rushed into the bathroom to check the tub, that's how real I felt it was. Of course Mark wasn't there. He was sleeping very peacefully in his bed. I never told him about the dream.

I couldn't think in terms of losing Mark. He had recovered from the great loss of blood from his circumcision at birth when things didn't look so good. When he was two, he had a severe case of hepatitis and the doctors in Boston told us he wouldn't make it. His body was yellow and his liver was so swollen that Mark's measurement at the waist was 30 inches. But he fooled the doctors at New England Medical Center and recovered fully. When he was four, he had a second bout with hepatitis, but once again recovered. He beat the pneumonia and the salmonella. Both times his chances seemed very slim to the doctors, and both times he won again. I had all the confidence in the world that Mark could continue to fight the AIDS. He was young, he loved to win, he had a positive outlook, and I filled his days with positive pep talks. I would never let it get him down. He had a healthy spirit.

On December 12, the junior high was having their annual International Foods Day. Mark decided to make petits fours. He loved to make desserts. He wore a paper mustache and a white hat. Mrs. Shelley Terry, a science teacher at the school, mentioned that day in an article she wrote in the CTL Newsletter entitled: "To Believe or Not to Believe." Her article was about trusting the doctors and believing that you could not catch AIDS through casual contact. She said that the real test for her came on International Foods Day. "Mark had prepared a colorful tray of petits fours. I selected a pink one and a green. I bought tea from the 'Chinese' delegation and returned to my desk for my next class would be arriving shortly. I arranged the 'goodies' before me and froze. I stared at them and remembered thinking how easy it would be, safer maybe, to just toss the little cakes into the basket. Do I really believe, or not? They were delicious."

On the night of my faculty Christmas party at the Biltmore in downtown Providence, Mr. Souza again took the boys out for a meal. This time they went to Boston and shopped at the Prudential Center and Copley Plaza. Mark came home with a Boston hooded sweatshirt. Scott came home with a Boston T-shirt.

We had many visitors all through December. Mark continued to have therapy for his ankle and soon he was just using one crutch. Gamma globulin was still being used to build up his immune system and he was still taking "chloro" for the salmonella.

Many relatives gave Mark money which he really appreciated. On Christmas Eve he received a large sum from Kathy and Joe

Swist. Mark was pretty wise in the use of money. He handled it well, but would spend it freely on baseball cards when he saw a bargain.

Mark didn't ask for much for Christmas. He was thrilled with his dirtbike and that was all he really wanted. We had already bought him the best helmet and goggles we could find as an early Christmas present. Even so we were able to give him other gifts which we knew he would be happy to have. He was very pleased with everything, but I really think he got more enjoyment giving the rest of the family the presents he had personally picked out for us. It was a pleasant Christmas for all of us.

The big excitement was that Mark could now put pressure on his ankle and was walking even if it was with a cane. The cane had belonged to my Grandfather LaBossiere with whom I was very close and it meant a great deal to me when Mark wanted to use it. It was a straight cane that tapered down toward the floor. Everywhere you saw Mark, you saw his cane.

Mark spent a great deal of time over the Christmas vacation working on his science fair project. He had done one in the seventh grade on hemophilia and won second prize. This made him eligible for the Massachusetts Region III Science Fair where he won a third prize. This year he chose to study the human eye.

As 1985 drew to a close, Mark's story was included in area media reports on the important happenings of the year. Bob Kerr of the *Providence Journal* in his end-of-the-year report said, "Locally, the story of the year came quietly and warmly from Swansea—that often rambunctious, rough-edged town that proved to be filled with class and caring as it rallied behind a young AIDS victim."

He went on to say, "The people of the town showed the kind of generous spirit and willingness to stop and think that was too often lacking to the north and south, east and west. In a year marked by the rush for easy answers, neatly wrapped feelings and the quick fix, Swansea provided the hopeful counterpoint. It opened up and showed itself special."

Mary Falvey, writing about the year in *The Spectator* said, "With genuine concern and an outpouring of compassion and support, Swansea students and parents rallied around a junior high student stricken with AIDS. The story made national news and Swansea was heralded as a community with a heart, its school superintendent for distinguishing himself in a responsible and courageous way." She went on to say that Mark "continues his education confident that he has the support of parents, peers, faculty and friends throughout town."

Joseph LaPlante of the *Providence Journal* also had an end-of-the-year story on Swansea with the headline: "'85 was year kindness beat fear of AIDS in Swansea." This large article covered the opening of school, the Swansea meeting, the Friends of Mark, and the dance. LaPlante said that Swansea was one of the nation's smaller towns, but "stood taller than nearly every city in America last fall when its residents showed compassion and understanding to a 13-year-old schoolboy stricken with AIDS."

As 1985 ended I had mixed emotions. I wondered what type of year 1986 would be for Mark and our family. I didn't think it could be much worse than '85 had been, but little did I know what was in store for us.

7

*"I'm strong and healthy today.
I'm a mean machine. And I'm going to
get better and better and better."*

—Mark Hoyle

The year was only a couple of weeks old when things began to crash. Literally. Mark's friend Marc Medeiros was selling his dirtbike because he bought a newer one. Scott was interested in looking at it. Marc's father told us he'd bring it over for Scott to try and we could let him know after Scott tried it out. He brought it over on a Saturday night.

The next day, right after church, we came right home so Scott could try the dirtbike. Dale thought we were in too much of a hurry, but Scott was very excited about the possibility of having a dirtbike of his own. He put on his helmet and gloves and heavy-duty shoes. Mark came out to watch us try it in the backyard. I was planning on teaching Scott just like I had done with Mark. We both got on the bike and I explained how to work the gas by moving the handlebar. We started off fine, but a little fast. As we approached the back of the yard we were supposed to turn and go back toward the house in an oval shape. Scott seemed to panic as we came to the turn. Instead of letting up on the gas, he gave it more gas and he didn't turn. It happened so fast that I couldn't do anything about it. We went straight and crashed right into the six-foot stockade fence. We both fell off and the bike came down on top of me. Luckily, Scott wasn't hurt. I was a nervous wreck worrying that he would have an internal bleed.

I ached all over. My thumb was all bruised, I had a small cut just above my eye, and my leg hurt. When I looked down at my leg, I noticed a big hole in my pants and a lot of blood. Mark hobbled out to us and Dale came running out. She had witnessed the whole scene from the sliding glass doors in the kitchen.

Dale was concerned for Scott, but he seemed fine. I told Dale that I was bleeding and she told me to get a bandaid for it. I said, "I think it's more serious than that." Mark wanted me to hold the spot with a clean handkerchief which I did. When I rolled up my pant leg, I noticed that it was a pretty deep gash. I told Dale she better drive me to the hospital and she said, "Come on, you can't be that bad!" I told her I thought I needed stitches and it would be best to have Scott checked out, too.

Off we went to St. Anne's Hospital. Mark stayed in the waiting room, while Dale went from room to room checking on Scott, Mark, and me. Scott was fine, I had 20 stitches!

That was it for the dirtbike. Scott said he never wanted to ride on one again. I was glad of that. Luckily the dirtbike wasn't damaged much and Drew took care of it for us. That afternoon, however, Mark still rode his dirtbike when he got home from the hospital.

Toward the end of the month, Mark started running slight fevers. Different medications were started, while others were dropped. On the 22nd we visited Dr. Smith in Providence. Mark's white blood count was 2.3 (2300) and his hemoglobin was 11.3. His platelets were 160,000. Because of his fevers, Dr. Smith wanted to see him again the following Wednesday.

Of course, on the 22nd, his temperature was 98.8 when we saw the doctor. The next day was fine, too. But Friday night it was 102.5 and 103.0 at 4:00 A.M. the next morning. He complained of a stiff neck that Saturday, too. His temperatures varied greatly from that day on: One hour it would be 99.0, then an hour later he would say, "I'm starting to get hot again" and his temperature would be 103.0.

On the 29th when we went back to see Dr. Smith, Mark's temperature was 101.0 at 6:45 A.M. and 98.6 at the time of his visit. His white blood count went down to 1.5 (1500) in one week's time and his hemoglobin also went down to 10.3. But his polys had gone up to 86. His lymphs went down to 10. There was no rhyme nor reason to his counts.

Mark hated having his temperature taken, but we wanted to watch him closely so we could prevent any serious illness before it got started. He continued to ride his dirtbike, go to movies, visit flea markets and card shops, and go to school. Some days we wouldn't let him go to school because of high temperatures.

The one good thing about January was that he didn't have any serious bleeds. Having a sore ankle limited his activities so much that he didn't have a chance to get hurt. He did receive seven vials of factor VIII for therapy.

Scott had a pretty good month, too. He only needed five vials for his right elbow and left knee. That damn knee was always giving him problems.

Another person having a good month was Superintendent McCarthy. On January 19, Bernie Sullivan, writing in the *Providence Journal*, devoted his whole column to Mr. McCarthy. He told how "a young boy named Mark, his family, a school system and a town are all richer" because of him. Mr. Sullivan told about the heat that Mr. McCarthy received from some, but he never backed down. Mr. McCarthy had this to say about the article: "This better not turn out to be a teary tale about how wonderful I am or I'm going to be mad. I'm no hero. Hell, the kid is the hero. And don't forget the school committee, the faculty, the kids in school and the people of this town. Those are the ones who deserve the accolades. Not me."

Mr. McCarthy received the prestigious President's Award from the Massachusetts Association of School Superintendents, Inc. It was in recognition of his leadership and the professional manner in which he handled the AIDS problem. This award also showed that the majority of school superintendents supported letting an AIDS victim go to school. Mr. McCarthy brushed off comments that his action was courageous, saying simply, "We did what we were supposed to do. The students' reaction in welcoming Mark is a tribute to the young man."

Mr. McCarthy was also named Citizen of the Year for 1985 by a unanimous vote. It is Swansea's highest honor. The committee had this to say about Mr. McCarthy:

We understand this decision to allow a Swansea child, who was stricken with AIDS, to continue his education in the school setting was not easily arrived at. We understand that Mr. McCarthy took a crash course on the subject. We acknowledge that he, by making this decision, also honored the power of education and the basic integrity of citizens of Swansea.

He lit the candle that dispelled darkness of fear and ignorance. Swansea can be proud that one of their own took this step forward in the best tradition of the people of the United States of America, where we stand for the victim and put our own lives on the line for our convictions.

The child has the right to an education, in this instance, is a bottom line. Mr. McCarthy's decision to stand for this right is a landmark not just in our town but for that right worldwide.

Besides being voted the Citizen of the Year, marking this heroism, it should also be noted that Mr. McCarthy's long career in education in our town has been a constantly forward movement, to give each year a better opportunity for every child of Swansea.

Indeed, Jack McCarthy did have a long career in education in Swansea. He started out as a teacher in town 30 years ago and worked his way up the ladder to principal, assistant superintendent, and since 1977, superintendent.

Although he doesn't consider himself a hero, Mr. McCarthy jumped into a river in 1966 and rescued a drowning boy who had stopped breathing. To our family, allowing Mark to attend school took more courage than his river rescue, and we will always consider him a "hero."

February brought more up and down temperatures for Mark. Thinking back on them now, he must have felt really lousy, but he never complained. I know that when I have an occasional temperature I feel terrible, and Mark had high temperatures many, many days.

Gamma globulin and therapy continued into February. On the 7th, I had to chaperone a dance at my school and my whole family went with me. Mark didn't have a good time because he wasn't feeling the best and he didn't know too many of my students. It was Catholic Schools Week and Father John Smith, the Director of St. John School, had surprised me earlier that day, when we had an assembly to thank everyone associated with the school. He called me up to the stage and had Maggie Cawston, the mother of one of my sixth grade students, come up too. She took the microphone and talked about my 17 years of dedicated service to the school. She presented me with a card that listed all the families who contributed to a gift certificate for a three-day visit to Cape Cod. This included spending money as well. Maggie and Linda Batchelder, another mother, had contacted the parents of the children to tell them of their plan. It was a beautiful recognition and it showed how much the school community backed my family. It was especially nice, since we hadn't taken a vacation in 1985, and the whole family really needed one.

Dale wrote a diary in February about Mark. Here is a week in his life as recorded in it:

Saturday, Feb. 8th, At 10 A.M. Mark had a temperature of 98.6. He felt great and went sledding with Scott and Becky Marchand. Later we all went duckpin bowling. At 4:00 P.M. he was still feeling great. His temperature was 98.8.

Sunday, Feb. 9th, At 9:00 A.M. Mark's temperature was 98.0. He felt good again. We went to church and then Mark went sledding. Later the boys wanted to go bowling again so we took them. He went to bed at 8:30 P.M.

Monday, Feb. 10th, Mark had a 98.0 temperature and felt good. He went to school and then went to the mall to "Just Fun" to play video games. He met his friend Dave Gorman there. He had a 98.0 temperature at night too, and went to bed at 8:30 P.M.

Tuesday, Feb. 11th, He woke up and felt hot. His temperature was 100.4. He took a shower and went to school even though he didn't feel the greatest. Gave him two tylenol. He felt better after school—99.8 temperature at 3:00 P.M. He rode his bike and shoveled driveway—then he took a nap. Sue came for therapy at 5:00.

Wednesday, Feb. 12th, He had a subnormal temperature. He felt good. After school he was out riding his bike—playing in the snow—did homework—stayed up a little later than usual that night.

Thursday, Feb. 13th, Woke up feeling a little warm, although his temperature was 99.4. Took shower, had one tylenol, seemed OK. Came home from school and went to "Just Fun" for two hours with Dave Gorman — ate good — went to bed at 8:30.

Friday, Feb. 14th, normal temperature — went to school feeling fine! Sue came at 5:00 for therapy — a good day!

The following week was vacation week. I had made reservations at the All Seasons Motor Inn which is in West Yarmouth, Massachusetts. It is also known as Bass River. Before we could go I had to drive up to Rhode Island Hospital to get some medication for Scott. He had a loose tooth and it kept bleeding and bleeding. Not too many people have ever stopped to think how ordinary minor problems like a loose tooth could be a major problem for a hemophiliac. Even going to the dentist can cause problems, or just brushing your teeth. Amicar is the medication that is given to hemophiliacs for mouth bleeds, along with the factor VIII.

We had a great time at the Cape. Mark was healthy and we went to many gift shops which the kids loved. We also visited a baseball card shop in Hyannis that had everything. Mark spent a lot of money there. The trip wasn't without problems. The first night at the motel the electricity went off just as everyone had changed into pajamas. A car had hit a telephone pole and we had no lights until around 3 A.M. when everything suddenly came back on.

The inn had a large pool, sauna room, jacuzzi, exercise room, and game room. The boys spent a good deal of their time using all the facilities. I knew that the AIDS virus could not be transmitted in a swimming pool, but I wondered to myself how many of the guests would still have gone swimming if they knew an AIDS victim was in the pool.

The National Seashore was a thrill for both boys with its massive sand dunes. We walked along the dunes and beach, although the weather was pretty cold.

Being a history teacher, I wanted to take the family to the Pilgrim Monument in Provincetown. The museum has something of interest for everybody and the granite structure has the best view of Cape Cod that there is. The only problem is, you have to climb the stairs and ramps to get to the top. But Mark wanted to do it, cane and all. It was excellent therapy for his bad ankle. The view from the top was breath-taking and Mark was happy that he decided to go up. It hadn't been an easy climb. There were many ice patches on the ramps where the heavy rain from the night before had frozen. But Mark always did like a good challenge. We climbed the 116 stairs and 60 ramps.

We drove all over the Cape from the tip at Provincetown on the east to Falmouth Harbor on the west. We stopped at all the Christmas Tree Shops that my wife could find. The important thing was that Mark was healthy. We all enjoyed our mini-vacation.

While our family was enjoying a Cape Cod vacation, Sue Travers and the Friends of Mark were busy at the Swansea Mall separating coins that were mixed with water, stones, and mud that had piled up in the wishing well there since 1975. The mall had decided to donate all the coins to the Friends of Mark.

Sue Travers was joined by two mothers and nine students who clawed, scraped, and dug their way through the large mounds of debris that had been shoveled out of the fountain by a maintenance man. Swansea Mall workers had also helped sort out the coins during their lunch breaks. The work took place in a back room at the mall.

They wanted to do as much as they could that week because the kids were on vacation from school. The group discovered that the banks wouldn't accept any of the pennies because they had turned green from being in the water. The Friends of Mark then sent the money to the Handicapped Workers Association in Weston, Massachusetts. In return for 15% of the total, they sorted out the coins and delivered them to the Treasury Department to be melted down.

The first small batch of coins produced $150. The two other mothers, Charlotte Oliveira and Katherine Medeiros, both parents of junior high students, said that they would continue to search through the coins until the whole project was completed.

Mrs. Oliveira is the mother of Joey, one of Mark's good friends. Mark had slept over at her house with her two boys and Joey had slept over at our house. They used to go to each other's birthday parties. Mrs. Oliveira commented to a reporter that, "I think it helps him emotionally. You can't help but love him."

Some of the students who volunteered to help were good friends of Mark, while others said they hardly knew him. One girl said, "I never even knew him, I just know I'm helping. If you have people helping that don't even know you, it makes you feel better." And I can say that we certainly agree with that girl whose name was Lisa Curry, age 13. Mark did really appreciate everything that was being done for him—by friends and strangers alike.

Debbie DeMaio gave us the name of a family in Longmeadow, Massachusetts, which was going through the same thing we were. Dale spoke on the phone many times with Suzanne White, but we never met the family in person. Gary and Suzanne's son Todd was a hemophiliac with AIDS-Related Complex. It was good therapy for both mothers to talk about their similar experiences.

Mark had another appointment with Dr. Smith during the vacation week. His white blood count dropped a little more to 1.4 (1400) and his hemoglobin also went down to 9.9. His polys went down, too, from 86 to 66, but his lymphs had gone up to 16. But Mark felt good. We didn't tell him about any of his blood counts. We wanted him to stay as positive as he could.

Mark started school again the following week. But Monday night he was sick with a 101.3 temperature. He didn't go to school Tuesday because he had a 102.5 temperature in the morning which increased to 103.0 in the afternoon even with Tylenol. (Hemophiliacs cannot take aspirin because it causes their stomachs to bleed.)

By Friday, Mark was feeling a little better, and went to school with his science project. I planned to meet him after school to give him a ride home because the judging was after school. Mr. Devine came out to the parking lot to get me. Mark felt sick again. He had already been judged, so it was good that he had lasted for that, otherwise all his work on it would have been wasted. Mark ended up winning third prize in the eighth grade. This qualified him for the Southeastern Regional Science Fair to be held at Bristol Community College in Fall River.

Mark had seven vials of factor VIII in February. Most were

for therapy, but he did have a knee and back bleed on the 27th and 28th. He was still just as good as the doctors at getting the treatment into himself on the first try all month. Scott had eight treatments for his left knee, right elbow, and his mouth.

Mark's knee continued to swell and cause him a lot of pain as we moved into March. In fact, he had to have treatment every day, sometimes twice a day for 12 straight days in March. We made an appointment with Dr. Lucas because we feared that the salmonella had come back and settled in his knee. Fortunately, this was not the case; it was just a bad bleed due to his hemophilia.

On Sunday, March 9, we celebrated Scott's birthday, although his birthday is actually the 10th. Scott had many of his friends over and we all went bowling. Other than the knee bleed, Mark was feeling great and went with us and bowled. The whole weekend we didn't take Mark's temperature because he was feeling great! Everyone had cake and ice cream back at our house. Toward the end of the party, Mr. Souza came over. He had taught most of the boys whom Scott invited. That night he stayed for supper and Mark and Scott began to call him "Uncle Dave."

Mark's blood counts continued to drop in March. He had three appointments with Dr. Smith and his white blood count went down to .8 (800). His hemoglobin dropped to 8.9. His polys went down to 38, although his lymphs went up to 50. His temperatures were on the high side all month with the highest being 104.0. Therapy and gamma globulin continued.

The regional science fair was held on Saturday, March 22, and Mark was judged that morning. He was planning on spending the whole day there, because they had a number of activities planned for the students, but he had to call home for a ride. He wasn't feeling well again.

The next day he was sick also. He had a bad headache and was dizzy. His temperature was 102.0. When we went to see Dr. Smith on the 26th, he decided to admit Mark to the hospital again. Dr. Smith wanted to see what was causing these fevers.

Mark ended up on the same floor in Potter I at Rhode Island Hospital. He was in room 2 again, his old favorite. All the same nurses were still there and all the familiar doctors who had treated him before. They came in teams—the Hemophilia Department, the Infectious Disease group, the Orthopedic Department, etc. Mark answered all their daily questions and even kidded with them. He especially got along well with all the young residents.

It wasn't an easy stay for Mark. He had to have a bone scan, a lot of blood work, and a spinal tap. The spinal tap was much more painful this time since Dr. Smith did it while Mark was awake. The last time it had been done while Mark was under anesthesia for one of his ankle operations.

All the tests proved negative. The doctors did not find out what was causing Mark's high fevers. The hospital stay was seven days—from March 26 to April 1. Dale and I stayed nights on an alternating basis as promised. Mark received many cards again. He especially liked the ones from his classmates.

While Mark was in the hospital, the testimonial for Mr. McCarthy was being held at the Swansea American Legion Post 303 in their hall on Ocean Grove Avenue. Mr. McCarthy received a standing ovation from the large crowd. When he finished his acceptance speech, he received another standing ovation.

Mr. McCarthy, who grew up in South Providence, Rhode Island, and graduated from Providence College, was also presented a silver Revere bowl from the school committee—Robert Paquette, James Carvalho, Russell Howarth, Eugene Rutkowski, and Steve Dzalio. The bowl noted Mr. McCarthy's long career in education. It also mentioned his extra-curricular activities as assistant football coach, baseball coach, head football coach, etc.

Massachusetts Congressman Barney Frank was there to praise Mr. McCarthy. State Senator John Parker brought the Golden Dome Citation. State Representatives Philip Travis and Joan Menard also presented citations to the superintendent. Selectman Chairman Donald Hyland presented a citation and Sue Travers gave Mr. McCarthy a plaque. Various other officials also honored him.

The Town of Swansea puts out an annual town report. The 1985 spring edition had this to say about our case: "The commencement of school in the fall of 1985 attracted national attention to Case Junior High School. The administration's decision not to exclude a student diagnosed as having AIDS from regular classes became the subject of national news coverage. The standard of behavior of the administration, faculty, and students of the school was exemplary and set a standard for the nation. The Town of Swansea was recognized by the entire nation as a community of compassion and understanding. This achievement is a tribute to all members of the school community who contributed to this accomplishment."

Mark was happy to be home again. The weather was getting nicer, and we prayed that Mark would stay healthy. We wanted him to be put on AZT, the experimental drug that the newspapers were saying was so promising. Dr. Smith called Boston and sent two letters in Mark's behalf, but Mark was refused because of his age. We kept trying, because we simply had to do all that we could to fight for Mark's life. But we were unsuccessful, and Mark never was allowed to take it. This made us very angry. Here was a drug that might help our son, and they wouldn't let us have it. It seemed so unfair!

In March, Mark had 17 treatments, mostly for his left knee. Scott had eight treatments for his mouth, left knee, and right elbow.

Even though Mark was home from the hospital, his temperatures continued to run high. The day after he came home, April 2, he was very thirsty and had a bout of shaking chills. His temperature was 102.2. He still had his gamma globulin treatment, however. The next day he still was home from school with a temperature of 102.6. He complained of being very thirsty again and had the chills. By the next day he was a little better, his temperature had gone down, but Friday came and it was back up to 101.4. Dr. Smith wanted to see him again and told us to give him treatment in case he needed to do another bone marrow test. But Mark felt better in the afternoon and Dr. Smith decided not to do it. Mark was put on prednisone to see if it would boost his blood counts. It did help his appetite somewhat, but his counts continued to fall.

Early Saturday morning, 3:30 A.M. to be exact, Mark woke us up because he felt hot again. His temperature was 101.1. He had the famous "night sweats" for which AIDS is noted. Many nights we would have to change his whole bed because he would sweat so much. But the next day he felt stronger and stronger as the day progressed. By 6:30 P.M. he was down to 99.3 and felt strong enough to go to his school play, *Annie*. Sarah Deston, a nice girl from Mark's class, had the leading role, and Mark was anxious to see the play. Jennifer Nahas was also in it along with many of Mark's friends and teachers. *Annie* was one of Mark's favorite movies. We had *Annie* on tape, and Mark watched it over and over. He loved the play just as much. "The sun will come out tomorrow," Sarah sang; Mark loved that song. It was a positive song, full of hope. But it made me sad, just like "That's What Friends Are For." Mark liked that song, too, because it benefited AIDS research.

On Sunday, April 6, Mark's temperature went down to 98.4. It would remain low for 18 days. Not that he felt perfect, because he didn't, but he went to school just about every day during that stretch of time. He was tired and took a nap every afternoon, but he still managed to go out and ride his dirtbike and have fun.

It was no wonder he was so tired. His white blood count went down to .7 (700) in April and his hemoglobin was 7.4. His polys were 78 and his lymphs 15. His platelets were even low at 83,000.

During vacation week Mr. Souza invited us all to go with him to Boston. During the winter he had taken the boys to the Cape, but this time they decided they wanted us to have some fun, too.

It was a nice sunny day, April 24, and we went to Quincy Market. The boys liked shopping for souvenirs and trying the various foods. Later we went to the top of the Prudential Center to see the view of the city. The boys especially liked the view of Fenway Park, the home of the Red Sox. Mr. Souza took a lot of pictures of the boys. Mark had his Swansea Little League All-Star cap on. He never went anywhere without it. Just about every outdoor picture we have of Mark shows him with a baseball cap on. Mr. Souza treated us to dinner and then we headed home.

The next day Mark woke up at 9:00 A.M. His temperature was normal, but he was tired, went back to sleep, and stayed in bed until noon. As the day progressed, his temperature rose and he had the chills. He continued to get worse each day and finally was put back in the hospital on April 28.

Dr. Smith had kept close watch on Mark. He had even made another house call in April to check on him and we had two appointments at the hospital with him. Therapy continued in April and Mark only needed five treatments. Scott needed nine for his left knee, right elbow, and left hip.

I mention these treatments only to give an idea of what it was like caring for two hemophiliacs. Our refrigerator was well stocked with factor VIII. It usually had more shelves filled with treatment than food. We had to mix our own treatment using needles that were provided in the kit. We would then draw it up into a syringe and make sure the bubbles were out. We would also have to draw up some normal saline in a smaller syringe. Using a butterfly needle, Mark or I would insert the needle into a vein. When we were first learning, we would often miss the vein, meaning additional needle sticks. Sometimes the veins would collapse right in the middle of giving the treatment. When this happened, we had to start all over again in a new spot with a fresh needle. It was also very painful. The factor VIII would go into some other cells and really irritate them. Sometimes it would even take four or five needle sticks before we got it in correctly. I hated to give it to them, but it was better than traveling to the doctor's office or hospital emergency room all the time as we used to do. We both did get better at inserting the needle. The sooner the treatment got into their system, the quicker it would go to work for them, so that was an additional reason for learning how to give it.

Mark was depressed about being in the hospital again. He was put in room 5 of Potter I this time. This was his fifth time in the hospital since coming down with AIDS.

Again the cards came in by the basketful. Visitors were always there to comfort him. He would still joke around with them and all the doctors and nurses. He was praying that the doctors would find out what was wrong with him this time. They did blood work and a spinal tap, but still couldn't find the cause of the high fevers.

Mark kept himself busy by working with colored salt. The hospital supplied the salt and the colored chalk and we supplied the containers. He would rub the colored chalk on top of the salt in paper plates. After mixing about eight or 10 different colors he would pour them into a glass container in layers to make beautiful, colorful creations. He gave most of them away but we managed to keep three.

He also liked creating designs on T-shirts and pillow cases. The hospital supplied pillow cases and the proper markers for the job and we supplied the shirts. Dale also got into the creative mood. She and Mark did the bulletin board in the corridor across from Mark's room. The one that was up had been there for months and we all got sick of looking at it.

After four days, Dr. Smith decided to let Mark go home. There was no sense in keeping him in the hospital when they couldn't find out what was wrong with him. It was Thursday, May 1, and Mark was happy to be home with his family and his animals.

On May 2, Mark went shopping with Dale and out to eat, but when he came home he didn't feel well and had a 103.0 temperature with the chills. The next day he felt well enough to go miniature golfing and shopping, but at night his temperature was 101.8. On Sunday we went to church and then to a flea market in search of baseball cards. We also went out to lunch and Mark felt good enough to rake the lawn when we got home. He said he had a pretty good day, his highest temperature was 100.8.

Because of his fevers, we wouldn't let Mark go to school. But he did feel better on Monday. Mark was able to help Dale with some yard work, ride his bike, and play catch with his brother. On Tuesday, May 6, his temperature was the best it had been in quite a while—98.2. He played ball with the kids down at the corner.

On the 7th of May we had an appointment with Dr. Smith. Mark's white blood count was the lowest I can remember. It was .5(500). His hemoglobin was also very low at 6.9. He didn't feel well and spent a lot of his time at home just lounging around on the couch. By Thursday night, however, his temperature was down again and he said he felt great. He went out to lunch with his mother and that night he went to the show with some friends.

On Sunday, May 11, Mark got a bad case of the chills and his fever climbed to 103.8. It stayed high and his neck started to bother him. By the 13th, you could see that his glands were starting to really swell. We brought him in to see Dr. Smith and

he was admitted to Rhode Island Hospital again. Dr. Smith was
actually going to let Mark go home with medication, but Mark
talked him into admitting him. It was a good thing because it
turned out that Mark was a very sick boy.

They put Mark in room 2 of Potter I and gave him a blood
transfusion. He looked terrible! It was the worst he looked
since coming down with AIDS. His neck was swelling more
and more and he didn't even look like Mark anymore.

Dr. Smith told us that whatever Mark had this time was
very, very serious and he might not make it. He brought me
up to an office on the second floor and I met with the whole
hemophilia team. They were quiet while Dr. Smith did most
of the talking. I was very upset that Dr. Smith was so pessimistic, but I kept my positive outlook. I was so glad that Dale
didn't come to this meeting. She would have been heartbroken.
Dr. Smith wanted me to tell Mark that this might be it. He told
me that everyone who was really sick had the right to know
when death was near. They might have things they need to say
to people before they die. He wanted to know if I was going to
tell Mark or if I wanted him to do it.

I told Dr. Smith that I didn't want him to mention this to
Mark at all. And I told him that I had no intention of telling
Mark either. If we told him, he would die. I didn't want him
giving up. He was a fighter. He was a positive thinker. He didn't
need these negative thoughts. I told Dr. Smith, "You're not
God! Only God knows when we're going to die. Even though
Mark is so sick, we all could be in a serious accident today and
be killed."

Dr. Smith agreed not to say anything to Mark. I was proud
of myself for standing up to him. Even though I considered Dr.
Smith a good friend, I thought he was too pessimistic in this
case, probably because he also dealt with children with cancer
and had seen a lot of premature deaths.

I told Dale what they had said to me. She asked me if I believed it. I told her that I had a great deal of faith in God and
everything would work out. She asked me if I cried when they
told me this. I told her that I hadn't, but that I really had felt
like doing so. I had been brought up to believe that boys didn't
cry. I hadn't cried since I was a kid. Besides, I had to be tough

for everyone. What would my family think if I suddenly started crying?

Dale asked me again if I thought that this might really be it. "Of course not!" I shot back at her. "Our Mark is one tough kid. He's going to beat this thing!"

Just to help out a little, I said a nine-hour novena to the Infant of Prague. I was still asking for a cure. We hadn't received one yet, but I was still positive that God would answer my prayers. I even had my class at school say the prayer to St. Jude every day. He is the saint of impossible cases.

The doctors decided that Mark's neck on the left side should be operated on. It was Mark who helped them decide. Our shy son was no longer shy. All the hospital visits had made Mark realize that you have to stand up and speak out for yourself if you want to get any place in this world. He told the other doctors how it was his idea to be admitted and how Dr. Smith was going to let him go home. When they talked about waiting a couple of days to be operated on, he told the head doctor of Pediatrics that he wanted to get operated on tomorrow. Later, Debbie DeMaio told us that the doctor was very impressed with Mark and his determination. It was the first time that anyone had ever seen someone tell this doctor what to do and actually get him to listen. But Mark was special. The doctor scheduled the operation for the next day.

Once again Dale and I had to make the long walk with Mark down to the operating room. Once again we kissed him and wished him good luck. This was his fifth operation and we felt so bad for him.

The doctors had told us it would only be a small incision. But it turned out they needed to go deeper than they thought and Mark ended up with a two and one-half inch scar on his neck. The right side of his neck also swelled, but not as badly as the left.

We took Polaroid pictures each day so we could compare his neck. He looked so swollen and deformed in the early pictures, but as the days went by, the swelling went down and Mark looked good again.

The test results from the operation came back. Mark had come down with another opportunistic infection, a very serious bacterial infection named mycobacterium avium intracellularus and Dr. Smith told us that there were not many cases of people recovering from it. On top of all this bad news, we also found out that he had another virus flowing through his body similar to mononucleosis.

There were drugs to treat his problems, but they hadn't helped others too much. There were also experimental drugs that Mark could take. We read all about the side-effects: One was that the urine, sweat, tears, and possibly hair and skin would turn orange. We talked it over with Mark and we all agreed he should try them.

Each day Mark had to take two lamprene capsules, three INH tablets, one ansamycin capsule, five ethambutal tablets, one pyridoxine tablet, one prednisone tablet, and one iron (ferrous sulfate) tablet.

It was easy administering the medication in the hospital because the nurses knew the proper times for each. Later when Mark recovered, it was quite a job keeping track of everything and making sure he took his pills at the right time. Some had to be taken with food. Mark had a real hard time taking them at first because he was so sick and didn't feel like eating. He would vomit them up and we'd have to start all over again. But he did get better each day. I stayed out of school because Mark was so seriously ill this time. I didn't go back until May 29. Mark had very high temperatures during this hospital stay. Many were at 104.0 and one even reached 105.0.

Mark also had to go through another bone marrow test. The fevers were a big problem. Every time he spiked a fever, the doctors would do blood work. Mark felt he was losing too much blood and also sleep. He talked Dr. Smith into eliminating this practice. They had been doing it for weeks and nothing was showing up in the blood anyway.

Mark also lost a lot of blood one night when one of his IV tubes came unhooked. He was sleeping and the blood was all over his bed before he felt wet and woke up in a panic. He was really scared according to Dale, who was staying with him that night. From that time on, he always wanted his tubes taped.

The experimental drugs finally came in on May 22. We were so happy that they were in and that they might help Mark. Mark had a temperature of 102.4 when he started them. He had been in the hospital for 10 days. His neck was definitely improved.

The junior high sent cards and posters. My school sent them, too. A banner stretched across two walls. Mr. Devine came to visit and always kept Mark well informed on what was happening in school. Some of Mark's teachers came to visit. Maureen Bushell, the school nurse, came frequently and always had a gift for Mark. Teachers from my school also came and a few parents from St. John's, too. Priests and ministers came by and all our relatives gave support. Dave Souza was there just about every day. He had bought tickets at the Providence Civic Center for the circus before Mark took sick. We were hoping Mark would be out of the hospital so he could go, but he wasn't.

Greg Gagne, the starting shortstop for the Minnesota Twins, called Mark. He is our cousin and had last seen Mark at our house in January before he started spring training. Mark used to write to him quite often, and every time he found a Greg Gagne baseball card he would send it to him and ask him to sign it. Greg's father Elmer was a good friend of mine when we were kids.

Even though Mark was still running high temperatures, Dr. Smith decided to let Mark go home. He could take the medication just as well at home, and now that they knew what Mark had, he could recover at home more comfortably.

Mark came home on Saturday, May 24. It was Memorial Day weekend. Dr. Smith still wanted to see Mark the following week on Wednesday, the 28th. That's why I stayed out of school until the 29th. I had to help Dale with all the pills, and Mark still was running high fevers. The day he came home he had a fever of 102.8.

Mark continued to feel lousy the rest of the month. His fevers reached 104.6 and we wondered if the experimental drugs would work.

I didn't have to give Mark any treatment in May, but he did receive some for his bone marrow test and operation. I did have to give Scott 11 treatments for his right elbow, his finger, and his left knee.

Meanwhile, the Friends of Mark were also keeping in touch with Ryan White's family in Kokomo, Indiana. In a newspaper article in the *Herald-News* in May, the headline read: "Friends

of Mark mount campaign for teen with AIDS in Indiana." Sue
felt bad for Ryan and was hoping she could get people to send
letters and cards to Ryan. She also asked people to write to the
school officials in Indiana.

Sue corresponded regularly with a family friend of the Whites,
Arletta M. Reith. Mrs. Reith told Sue, "I have tried to get financial help for Ryan's family, but to date I have gotten 10 letters.
There are Kokomo people who actually hate Jeanne (Ryan's
mother). That's so sad because Ryan's family has virtually no
support here. You are to be commended for your efforts there."

Mrs. Reith continued in her letter, "I don't care to have small
time terrorists calling me on the phone, threatening me. Maybe
some people here don't care they live in a city with that kind
of image, and maybe some rationalize it away, by saying it's
none of the rest of the country's business. But it's an image
nonetheless, whether it's right or wrong. We have to do something about the image."

I can only say that having the support Swansea gave to Mark
really, really helped. I don't know how we all would have gotten
through all this without it. Sue Travers thinks that God was
behind her all the way. Everything fell into place too easily for
it to be otherwise, she said.

I only hope and pray that people will listen to their doctors
and start treating all AIDS patients with the love and understanding that is needed so very much. They are all human beings and need to be treated as such.

The Friends of Mark had some money in their bank account
and they asked Mark if there was anything they could buy him.
He said that the only thing he really wanted was too expensive.
They asked him what it was and he said, "A video camera."

They found a fine one on sale and bought it for him. Mark
was thrilled. We read all the directions together and then tried
it. At first we weren't working it right, but finally we got the
knack of it. Mark took pictures of our family, our cats, and his
room. He loved it, though it was very heavy on his shoulder.
The Friends of Mark solved that problem by giving him a tri-
pod. I tried to use the camera as much as possible to take pictures of Mark.

The first week of June was a busy one for Mark. On the 2nd,

he had to go for X-rays for his lungs at Charlton Memorial Hospital in Fall River. This was where my sister worked. Dr. Mucciardi had sent us for X-rays just to make sure that everything was still fine. It had been a year since his pneumonia. On the 3rd, Debbie DeMaio came for a visit and on the 4th, we had Nancy Keyes come for his gamma globulin treatment. Sue Gemma came at night for therapy. On the 5th, it was a visit to Dr. Mucciardi's office and on the 6th, it was his cousin Matt's birthday party.

Although the week was busy, Mark still wasn't feeling well. We kept a record of his temperatures on a chart and that week he peaked at 105.2. I also would write down how his days were. On June 1, I had written down "poor—all day." On the 2nd and 3rd, I had him as "fair." Wednesday was the day his temperature shot up to 105.2. It was 3 o'clock in the afternoon and it scared us all to see it go so high again. By Thursday his temperature was down to 103.2 when he woke up. It continued to go down as the day went on. I ended up writing "good day" on my chart.

It was a beautiful June day and I decided to take Mark's picture on the video camera. As he walked around the deck in the backyard he said, "I'm strong and healthy today. I'm a mean machine! And I'm going to get better and better and better." He then climbed up his ladder and went in his tree house and started doing a little dance. He always liked to clown around for the camera. I told him, "You have a lot of energy today, considering you had a 103.0 temperature this morning."

"That's right. Positive thinking!" he responded. Later he climbed down and walked to his brother's clubhouse in another tree. I walked behind him with the camera on. He still had a limp, but he was walking much better. Excellent—when you think the doctors had said he might not ever walk again.

Friday, the 6th, was a "good day" and Saturday was "very good." He went to the mall with some friends to play video games.

During the week he also rode his bicycle for the first time since coming home from the hospital. "This is fun," he said on the video camera. Dave Souza came over and we taped him, too. All our friends and relatives were anxious to see themselves on television.

On Sunday, June 8, Mark was sick again. He felt very tired

all day. But by Monday, he felt better, even though he did have a 102.0 temperature. He had been wanting a new dog. I guess he missed Cleo. We tried to talk him into getting a small dog, but he insisted he would really like a big one like a German shepherd. When I came home from school, Mark was sitting on the park bench on our front deck with a puppy on his lap. It was a German shepherd!

"Where did he come from?" I asked.

"Mom and Nana Hoyle took me to Fall River to look for a puppy. We were supposed to be just looking," he responded. "And I'll tell you the whole story. . . . "

So here is the story of the new addition to the Hoyle family as told by Mark: "I wanted to go out today because I was feeling good. So I said to Mom, 'Why don't you call Nana Hoyle and see if she can take us to the Animal Rescue League?' So she said, 'OK,' but Nana wasn't home. The next thing you know the doorbell is ringing and it's Nana Hoyle. What a break! I said, 'Hey Nana, I'm feeling good, how about driving us over to the Animal Rescue League and just look?' But Nana said, 'Well, I just came from Fall River, I wouldn't want to drive all the way back there and find nothing. So I'll call Papa and see if he can call Mike to see if they have any puppies.' So Papa called Mike and then he called us back. They had some so we went over there. When we got there Mike had this little puppy, right here (pointing to Chipper), this little guy right here, on the counter waiting for us. So my mom said, 'We're just looking today.' And then Mike said, 'Oh, no, you're not, this is YOUR dog!' So we took him home and here he is. See how he comes to me. He really likes me. This dog and I are going to be great friends."

Later that day I got a call from Dr. Smith. He asked me if I would do him a favor and talk to this friend of his from California who was writing about the "Swansea case." I told him I would be glad to.

David L. Kirp is a professor of law and public policy at the University of California, Berkeley. He makes his home in San Francisco. He was planning to write about Mark and then have the story published in some national magazines.

We welcomed him to our home and he talked to all of us on our screened-in patio. Mark wanted me to take some video scenes of David. It was the first interview we had granted since Mark Patinkin's article.

We all liked David and became instant friends. Later we kept in touch through phone calls and letters. He sent Mark a whole box full of baseball items from California, including an autographed ball signed by Dave Kingman. It had T-shirts, yearbooks, calendars, stickers, and baseball cards.

The rest of the week Mark was pretty good, although he had a high temperature every day. The highest all week was 102.8.

Ron Devine called me to see how Mark was doing. He asked me if Mark was well enough to go to school for the last day on Friday, the 13th. I told him that if he was well enough, I would certainly drive him in for the assembly which he wanted Mark to attend. I had a hunch that he was planning to give Mark some kind of recognition.

I asked Mark if he wanted to go to school the last day to say good-bye to his friends. He was very excited that I thought he was well enough to attend. He was worried that he would get sick, but I told him that his mother and I would wait out in the car. He could come out any time. We planned on doing some reading while we waited.

At 7:00 A.M. that Friday, Mark's temperature was 99.4. He said that he felt great. He took a shower, had a good breakfast, and we drove him to school. Ron Devine had told me at what time the assembly would start, so we arrived about 15 minutes early so he could go to his homeroom with his class.

Ron had told me that Dale and I were both welcome to go to the assembly, but Mark didn't want to be the only student with his parents there so we didn't go in. I'm sorry now we didn't. And I'm sorry now I didn't bring the video camera. It was a very special moment in Mark's life. Mr. Devine was giving out various awards for different subjects. He saved the best for last. The Principal's Award was handed out annually to a deserving boy and girl. Mark told us later how Mr. Devine talked about what a hero is and how Case Junior High had their own hero; it was Mark! He told us later that he couldn't believe his ears when his name was called. The whole student body and faculty stood up and gave him a thundering ovation as he made his way, limping, to the front of the media center. School nurse

Maureen Bushell told us later that his classmates "just went wild. It was the most thunderous applause I have ever heard," she said. Faculty and students alike continued to clap while Mark made his way up to the stage. The applause stopped for a minute while Mr. Devine presented Mark with his award, but then it started up again as he made his way slowly back to his seat.

Dale and I, sitting in our car near the door, could hear the applause. I had thought I heard Mark's name called out. I told Dale that they were cheering for Mark. We felt so happy for him.

When Mark came out to the car, he walked right up and got in and acted like nothing at all had happened. Then he yelled out, "I got the Principal's Award! Everyone gave me a standing ovation! It was wonderful!" That was one of Mark's favorite words, "wonderful."

Mr. Devine came out to shake Mark's hand one more time and to tell us about the loud applause. He said everyone there was so pleased that Mark could make it. He looked so good. We told Mr. Devine that we could hear all the applause from our car. He was disappointed that we hadn't actually witnessed it. But it was Mark's special moment, a moment in time that he would treasure for the rest of his life. Many times that summer he spoke to us about how special his classmates had been. For the whole school to back him like that was simply amazing. Over and over he would talk to us about that special day when he received the Principal's Award.

8

"I think it was the hardest that I had ever prayed in my life. I begged God to heal Mark. I asked Him to give me the AIDS and take it away from Mark."

—Jay Hoyle

Saturday Mark was feeling good. His temperature was 98.6 when he woke up at 9:00 A.M., but it went up slowly during the day to 101.0 by 6:00 P.M. We hoped that he would be healthy for Sunday. It would be Father's Day and we had plans to go to Fenway Park to see the Boston Red Sox.

Paul Scanlan of Attleboro, Massachusetts, had arranged the whole day. I had three of his children in my classes at school and Paul had written to me earlier about his idea of treating Mark to a game. We had to wait until Mark was healthy enough to go. Paul hired a limousine and arranged for front row seats next to the Red Sox dugout. But the best part was that he had also arranged for us to go out on the field and meet many of the Red Sox players personally. We called the day, "Mark's Day," but it was a treat for our whole family. It was especially nice that it was Father's Day. I had memories of last year's special day when I spent it at the hospital with Mark. Things looked so gloomy then, but Mark had recovered. He was such a fighter. It had been a tough year, but he was up for the fight.

The sun was shining when we woke up and I hoped everything would go well. The boys both wanted to wear their Red Sox shirts and baseball caps. Mark wore a blue shirt with his blue cap and Scott wore a red shirt with his red cap. They both wore white pants and sneakers.

As they sat waiting on the park bench on our front deck, I videotaped them. This is what Mark said on camera: "Hello, this is the day that we go to see the Boston Red Sox in a limou-

189

sine. It is called 'Mark's Day.' Isn't that wonderful! And we're going to be eating donuts and other pastry in the limo. I'm sure it will have a TV and stuff like that. Gee, this sure is an exciting day!"

The gray limousine arrived right on schedule and the driver, Tom Broderick, owner of the Great Woods Limousine Service, was all spruced up in a black tux. He opened the doors for us and showed us to our seats. We weren't used to such royal treatment. The limousine had a color TV, VCR, stereo, refrigerator, etc. Dale and I had coffee and Danish, the boys had orange juice with their treats.

When we arrived at Fenway, we were dropped off right at the gate. Mr. Broderick escorted us right to the entrance where Mark and Scott received baseball gloves with the Red Sox insignia on them — a right-handed glove for Mark and a left-handed one for Scott. It was Kool-Aid Glove Day and all the youngsters would be receiving one. A Red Sox public relations official met us and escorted us right down onto the field. We had been to this beautiful ball park before, but never dreamed of going out on the field.

I videotaped everything with Mark's camera. The Red Sox were taking batting practice and the park was practically empty. They hadn't opened up the gates yet. The first person we were introduced to was Bob Montgomery, a Red Sox announcer and former catcher. The boys asked him for his autograph and he was glad to give it. Mark had baseball cards of Bob at home and he was sorry he hadn't brought them to be signed. But I told him we probably wouldn't have the time to go searching for each player's individual card. Besides, he could always send the cards by mail if he wanted them autographed.

The next person we met was Roger Clemens. Mark had listened to his 20-strikeout game when he was in the hospital back in April. He wasn't able to watch it because it was on a cable channel. Scott and I saw the tail end of it when we got home from the hospital that night. The boys talked to Roger about the terrific season that he was having. He made some small talk and then Mark asked him if he could have his autograph. Roger was glad to sign his name for both boys in Mark's book. He was very friendly with the boys and posed for some still pictures which Dale was taking.

The boys also met Bob Stanley, Mike Stenhouse, Sammy Stewart, Rich Gedman, Mike Brown, Johnny Pesky, Dave Stapleton, Joe Sambito, Ed Romero, Joe Morgan, John McNamara, and Don Baylor. All of them signed their names twice, one for each boy. Joe Sambito even went into the clubhouse to get the boys each a shiny new official American League ball which he signed. Joe wrote: "To Mark, I enjoyed meeting you at Fenway. Joe Sambito 6/15/86." He wrote the same on Scott's ball.

Our guide even took us in the Red Sox dugout. It was a big thrill for me to sit in it, too. When Mark asked the manager, John McNamara, for his autograph, he said, "Hey, John, could I please have your autograph?" It sounded like he had known him all his life. I was surprised that he didn't say "Mr. McNamara." But Mark and I had watched every game that we could for years and years and we almost felt like we knew the players personally. Mark was a little disappointed that we didn't get to meet a few of his idols like Tony Armas, Dwight Evans, and Wade Boggs. But they had taken batting practice earlier and had already gone back into the clubhouse.

As game time approached, we made our way to our front row seats. We watched as Wade Boggs and Dwight Evans warmed up right in front of us. This delighted Mark and Scott. The players also had to pass right by us as they made their way to the on-deck circle. The boys took pictures of them as they passed and I taped parts of the game on the video camera.

But it was very hot and we were sitting right in the sun. Mark started to feel sick. Dale rubbed his back with some ice from a soft drink to cool him off, but it didn't help. I took Mark into the shade under the seats and he vomited. I thought he might feel better after this, but he didn't and so we eventually had to leave. It was the fifth inning. We didn't miss too much anyway, Milwaukee won the game.

The air-conditioned limo and a cold soda helped Mark feel better again. He felt bad about having to make the whole family miss the game. But I reminded him that the best part was meeting the players and actually being on the field and in the dugout with the manager, coaches, and players. I told him it was a perfect Father's Day for me because the Red Sox had been my favorite team since I was a child. And I had never dreamed that I would ever be walking on the field at Fenway where my idols played! And to sit in the Red Sox dugout with the players was just unbelievable!

Mark was happy that I was happy. He would do anything to make us happy. I felt bad for him that he couldn't have enjoyed his special day a little better. I asked God why He couldn't let Mark feel well for the entire day. Of course, I didn't get an answer.

I called Paul Scanlan as soon as we arrived home to let him know that Mark really enjoyed the day and to thank him for everything that he had done for our family.

Mark's temperature, which had been 101.8 in the morning before we left, fell to 97.8 at 8:00 P.M. that night. The next day Mark felt super and we played catch in the backyard. Dale taped Mark with the camera. Mark wanted her to stand right behind my shoulder so it would look like the ball was coming directly at the camera. At the end of the day I wrote "very good day" on his temperature chart.

On Tuesday we had to take Mark to Charlton Memorial Hospital because Dr. Mucciardi wanted a gallium lung scan done. They injected the dye that day and we would return on Thursday for the X-rays. We asked if they could also check out his ankle. It seemed that during therapy on the 13th, Mark heard something snap and it was getting more and more painful every day. We had been giving the factor VIII every day, but it wasn't getting any better.

Wednesday, June 18, was my birthday. I turned 39 and I was much happier than I had been a year earlier when Mark was so sick. Mark was feeling great except for his ankle. We had an appointment at Rhode Island Hospital with Dr. Rosenfield, a hematologist who was filling in for Dr. Smith while he was away. Mark's white blood count was up to 1.6 (1600). That was the highest it had been since January 22. His hemoglobin was up to 7.9 and things looked like they were improving. Dr. Rosenfield thought Mark's problem was an ankle bleed and not an infection.

On Thursday Mark had his X-rays. He had been through the procedure before so he knew what to expect. He had to stay in one place without moving for a long period of time as the camera scanned him. Then he had to move to a different position for another long period. After many positions and many pictures, Mark was finally finished and we left.

The next day Mark had his gamma globulin treatment. He didn't feel well in the morning, but came to life in the afternoon. I was asked to be a chaperone at Scott's teacher's pool party. Mrs. Friar annually invited her entire class to swim in her in-ground pool and to feast on hot dogs, hamburgers, and other good treats. I brought Mark's camera (with his permission) and taped the proceedings. Then we all watched it on Mrs. Friar's VCR. Later that day I made a copy for her.

Meanwhile Mark was on crutches because he couldn't put any pressure on his sore right ankle. It didn't stop him from doing things, however. He was feeling healthy, and that was the main thing. He went to the mall on Saturday and then we all went to a dance recital at night. Linda Nahas and Sharon Marchand asked me to tape the show because their daughters were both in it. It was the same dance troupe that had danced for Mark at Swansea Mall and both boys were anxious to see the girls again. I taped the whole show and then made a copy for them. On Sunday Mark went to a movie.

The ankle continued to give him problems so we made an appointment with Dr. Lucas again. He felt that the problem was that some adhesions had pulled apart or snapped in the ankle during therapy. It was a bad bleed, but he did not think it was an infection. Mark was so relieved that he didn't have to have the ankle tapped again. Dr. Lucas also told us that the ankle was slowly fusing together. This meant that the joint would be "frozen" and would not move; it would be like one solid bone. Once the fusion took place, which could take months, it probably would end, once and for all, all the pain and bleeds. We wondered if this process could be speeded up. I guess an operation could have been done, but why put Mark in the hospital again?

At 10 P.M. that night, Mark's temperature shot up to 103.0. But by the morning, he felt good again and we took a ride down to Cape Cod.

I was out of school for the summer and taking my second summer off so I could spend more time with Mark. My class had sung "That's What Friends Are For" in honor of Mark at

their graduation. It brought tears to my eyes as I thought back
to how very sick he was the year before.

Mark was in his glory at the Cape. He loved gift shops and
he loved the baseball card shop in Hyannis. The highest his
temperature reached that day, June 24, was 98.8. As Mark
searched for cards he needed, Scott bought some Boggs and Yaz
cards. He was trying to get every card issued on both players.

Debbie DeMaio came for a visit on Wednesday. Mark had
another super day. I told her about calling Father William Babbitt, the healing priest. She thought it was a good idea.

Father Babbitt had been a brother of Holy Cross. He was my
Latin teacher at Monsignor Coyle High School in Taunton,
Massachusetts. Not too long after I had graduated, he had left
the order to become a priest. I always had liked him as a teacher
and a nice human being. He was a pleasant guy who was always cracking jokes. All the guys at school called him "Rex."

Many of the mothers of my students at St. John's had told
me that I should take my boys to see Father Babbitt. It seems
that Father Babbitt one day heard a voice that said, "Through
these hands, I shall work wonders," and from that day on he
was given the power to cure people. Folks flocked from all over
to attend his monthly healing service on Sunday afternoons
and his weekly prayer services during the week. I decided that
I would like to take the boys.

I called Father Babbitt and told him all about Mark having
AIDS and both of them having hemophilia. We arranged for a
private meeting at the rectory. Dale wasn't sure if she wanted
to come, but I talked her into it.

It was June 26, a Thursday, and the boys asked me why we
were going to see a healer. Did he really have the power to cure
them? I told them how many people have been cured by God.
I told them about Father Babbitt's healing power, but I didn't
tell them how most of the people he touched were "slain in the
Spirit." I made it quite clear to them that God doesn't heal
everybody, but it wouldn't hurt to try.

For those who have never heard the expression "slain in the
Spirit," or seen it in person, it is incredible! Father Babbitt, after
saying a beautiful mass, would have the congregation stand in
a straight line on the side of the church. Ushers would bring
up each row so that the entire proceedings were done very or-

derly. He would then place his hands on the head of a person and the person would drop to the floor as if he or she had fainted. Ushers would stand behind each person as Father Babbitt prayed over them and they would catch the people as they fell. The ushers would then gently lay them on the rug. It was amazing to see. People would just drop and they were all over the floor. By the time Father Babbitt reached the end of the row, most had awakened and had been replaced by more faithful. He would then work his way back down the row skipping over the people who were still lying on the floor. Some would be out for quite some time, while others would be out only a few minutes.

We met with Father in a private room and talked about old times. He joked with all of us and I could tell that Dale and the boys really liked him.

Soon he said that he was ready to pray over us. He asked me to stand behind Mark. Mark stood up in the middle of the room with his wooden crutches. Father Babbitt stood up with his metal ones for he had recently had surgery on both hips. Father Babbitt began to pray and he put his hands on Mark's head. Mark closed his eyes and seemed to go into a kind of trance. It seemed like he was sleeping. He didn't fall, but his crutches kept him up. Father Babbitt told us that he was "slain in the Spirit." "Isn't it beautiful," he said, "Mark is completely at rest."

I don't think Scott, who was sitting on the couch, knew what to make of it. Mark stood there for quite some time before he blinked his eyes a few times and then seemed to wake up. He sat down on the couch and then Father prayed over Scott. The same thing happened to him. Scott's eyes closed and he seemed like he was in a deep sleep. I was right behind him and he was swaying a little bit, but he didn't fall back. He was like this for a long time before he came out of it. It was not as though they were imitating behavior they had seen before. They had not known what to expect when they walked in.

Next Father prayed over Dale as I stood behind her. She did not get "slain in the Spirit." He asked me to come to her side and his hands touched my head. I could feel a surge of energy or power or something come into my head and I felt a little funny, but I fought the feeling. I did not fall back or go into any type of trance either.

Father Babbitt then talked to us some more and told us how he had suddenly received his powers from God. Then he told us how shocked he was the first time he started praying over people and they started falling all over the church like dominoes. I asked him why Dale and I didn't fall or be "slain" like the boys, but he said some people don't respond. One lady had been going to his weekly prayer service for over a year and had never been "slain." One young girl, he told us, usually was out for almost an hour. He invited us to go to one of his healing services. God works wonders at these North Attleboro services, he told us.

I had heard the stories of some of Father Babbitt's cures. I should say the Holy Spirit's cures because Father Babbitt always says that he is just an instrument of God. God is the Healer! My mother even knew a sister from Catholic Memorial Home in Fall River who was cured of cancer of the mouth. The doctors had announced no hope, but Father Babbitt prayed over her and she was cured. The cancer disappeared. The doctors couldn't believe it, but it happened.

I told Father Babbitt that we would see him at his next healing service. He said he was happy that we would be attending. He would also schedule another private service if we wanted. There was no charge for this.

The next day Mark was still running a 101.2 temperature and felt very tired. But he still wanted to go to the circus. Rosemary Baker from the "Wish Come True" organization had called to tell us that she had free tickets for all the members. The Clyde Beatty-Cole Brothers Circus was in New Bedford, Massachusetts. We had to make a sign for our front windshield that said "Wish Come True." Then we could park right next to the entrance. This was a big help for us since Mark was on crutches with his sore ankle.

We met Rosemary at the gate and were introduced to some other members. Soon we were all placed in reserved seats at center ring. The ringmaster welcomed all the members of the "Wish Come True" group. The boys enjoyed the show very much.

Saturday and Sunday were fair days for Mark. Usually his temperature was higher in the morning and would go down slowly during the day. He was still taking the great variety of pills for the mycobacterium avium intracellularus. He would go in the pool on nice days and help around the house. He played "Atari," spent a lot of time with his dog and cats, and continually read his baseball card magazines. He was always sending for an order somewhere or sending for an autograph.

On the last day of June we took Chipper for his shot. He was getting bigger and stronger every day. I was beginning to think that Dale had brought home a horse instead of a dog. Mark didn't feel well in the morning, but by afternoon his temperature was down to 98.0.

Mark had received 15 vials of factor VIII in June. One was prophylactic for therapy and all the rest were for his sore right ankle that continued to bother him. Scott, meanwhile, had a worse month. He needed 23 vials of treatment for his left knee, right ankle, right elbow, and large bruise on his buttocks. It seemed like all I did was mix treatment and give it to them. Between that, and keeping track of Mark's temperature and pills, it was a tough month.

July 1 was a bright and sunny day, and Mark wanted to help me complete a section of deck. He went with me to Grossman's to pick out the lumber and nails and helped me load it into the car. We liked working together on outdoor projects and he was a big help with nailing the boards in place and staining the wood. July 1 was also the day that Dr. Smith returned from vacation. We were happy that he would be around if we needed him. We had an appointment scheduled for the next day.

Wednesday, July 2, was a good day for Mark. The highest temperature he had was 100.2 and he told Dr. Smith that he felt "great." His white blood count dropped a bit to 1.3 (1300), but his hemoglobin remained the same at 7.9. His red blood count had gone up from 2.63 to 3.28. We were pleased with most of his blood counts, although we wished they were a great deal higher.

July 2 was also the last day he needed treatment for his right ankle. The swelling had gone down and he could put his weight on it again. He was still on the crutches for support because the ankle was still fusing.

July 3 was a "very good day." Mark was able to play catch with his brother despite the bad ankle. They loved playing whiffle ball in the backyard or in the driveway. They also would play with the tennis ball down at the corner. In the backyard they played "Home Run Derby." You either got a home run, which was on the roof of the house or over it, or you were out. This was a good game for Mark because he didn't have to run after the ball. Someone was always willing to shag the home runs when Mark was in the field. Mark could pitch and bat with no problem. He especially liked to bat. He had no problem hitting the ball for a home run either. I didn't think it looked too difficult to do until I played with them. I found out it is a lot harder than it looks.

The 4th of July would be special for us this year. Holidays always stick out in my mind and we all remembered how we had spent last year's 4th watching the fireworks from a St. Anne's Hospital window. This year Mark was feeling super and we made plans to go to the fireworks in person. Mark had plenty of company because we met his cousins and sat together on blankets to watch the display. Mark really enjoyed being there.

Saturday and Sunday Mark had poor mornings, but felt good enough in the afternoon to go swimming in our backyard pool. Monday was gamma globulin day and Mark felt great. He worked on his tree house, adding pieces of stockade fence to the sides. Now it looked more like a fort. He also went swimming again.

On the 8th of July, Mark had an appointment with Dr. Mucciardi. His appointment was at 2:00 P.M. His temperature at that time was 99.0 and the doctor was pleased with Mark's progress. Mark had even gained some weight since his last visit a month ago. To cap it off, his lungs sounded perfect. It was all good news.

Around this time, someone sent us a copy of *Education Daily*. The June 25th edition had an article about Swansea and Mark. "AIDS: Impact On The Schools" was the title with a heading of "Swansea, Mass.: How One District Dealt With An AIDS Case."

"It would be nice if for every horror story about AIDS in the schools, there were a success story to balance it," the article stated. "Well, there isn't, but there is one story that should give heart to school administrators looking with trepidation to the day they may have to deal with a student or employee with AIDS. That tale involves citizens of the southeastern Massachusetts town of Swansea, population 15,000, who rallied behind a Case Junior High student with hemophilia who caught AIDS from contaminated blood products."

The article went on to tell Mark's story including the great support of the Friends of Mark. It was a four-page report. Around the same time we also came across David Kirp's article in the *Christian Science Monitor*. He entitled it: "A Community tries to be caring."

"Mark is the kind of student whom commencement speakers extol as 'the promise of the future' or 'America's greatest asset,'" wrote David Kirp. "Last month he graduated from Case Junior High School in Swansea, Mass., where he had been on the honor roll, won prizes at the science fair two years running, and was a Little League all-star. But what makes Mark unique is this: He is the first child with AIDS who has been allowed to attend public school."

Mark was pleased to read an article about himself in a national publication. He always talked about how he wanted to be famous some day. I'm sure he could have been more publicized, if we had let him. But we wanted to protect him from the press so he could lead as normal a life as possible under these harsh conditions that he faced daily.

David Kirp ended his article by saying that, "What Swansea did has made Mark feel better about himself. And to hear the townspeople tell it, they feel happier about themselves, too. 'Isn't it something!' they kept repeating, pleased with how things have turned out. Swansea can teach the rest of the country a thing or two."

Wednesday, July 9, was an excellent day for Mark. In the morning he was strong enough to play baseball with the gang at the corner. Later in the afternoon I took pictures of him in the backyard with the video camera. Then I went in the pool and Mark came in, too, but stayed in his rubber boat with oars. I told him that he was too chicken to come in the water because it was so cold. Mark replied that he wasn't chicken and rowed over to the ladder. He stepped out of the boat and sat on the top step of the ladder. He put his feet in the water and complained to me about the "ice-cold" temperature of the water.

I told him to jump right in. But he asked me how long it took for me to get in. I answered, "About a second."

"Oh, no!" he laughed, "I didn't see you jump right in!" Meanwhile, Dale took video pictures of the two of us. Scott was over at a friend's house.

Mark inched his way down into the water and yelled, "Pain! Pain!"

I said, "Come on, Marky, don't be chicken on the camera." Mark laughed and made all kinds of excuses why he couldn't go in yet. I said, "Come on Mark, I've been in here for about a half an hour."

"I doubt it!" he yelled out and laughed. "Try five minutes!"

I told him that in less than a month, he was going to be 14. He wouldn't want any of his friends to see the tape that his mom was shooting—he would be embarrassed.

I swam over to the ladder and pulled him into the pool. Then I carried him across to the other side.

"You mama!" Mark yelled and laughed. "You're rotten! He's a mama," Mark told Dale. He was laughing and having a good time. I rubbed his back with the cold water.

"You're a mama!" he repeated.

"I thought you liked backrubs," I said.

"Not with cold water!" he responded. Then he leaned over and gave me a big hug and kiss on the cheek.

Mark continued to ride his dirtbike on all the days he felt well. Marc Medeiros would usually ride with him. And Mark never passed up an opportunity to go somewhere. Dave Souza took the boys to see Doug Henning perform his magic in Providence. Mark was really impressed. The next day he wanted me to go up in the attic to see if his magic tricks were still there. They were, and he practiced them until he was a "pro."

The next few days were excellent ones for Mark. He was in a great mood. He always had a smile on his face. We went miniature golfing and he played ball with the kids in the neighborhood.

But by Saturday, he was sick again and complaining of a stiff neck. His temperature was 101.8 and he spent the day on the couch. Dr. Smith started Mark on Motrin for the pain.

On Sunday there was a healing service in North Attleboro. Mark had a 103.3 temperature, felt itchy all over, and was just plain miserable. But he insisted that we take him to see Father Babbitt again.

Carol Hilsman, the mother of three of my former students,

met us in the parking lot and sat with us. This was our first public healing service and we were shocked at the size of the crowd. The church was completely filled. There were all ages present. The mass started and I was deeply touched by the way Father Babbitt said it, and the way the congregation responded. I can't really explain the unique way it was done, but one could feel a great sense of love in the air. There was a feeling of great holiness.

All the people held their hands up above their heads and sang praises to the Lord. They joined hands at times and formed a human chain that stretched from Father Babbitt at the altar to the back row of the church.

Father's sermon was very inspirational, but also laced with jokes thrown in at just the right time. Mark and Scott joined in with everyone else and seemed to enjoy the service.

After the mass, the healing service began. Ushers directed the people from the front pews to stand along the side. The rest of the congregation was singing, but my family was more interested in watching Father Babbitt. It was unbelievable to see these people "slain in the Spirit." I wondered if I would go out when it was my turn.

When our row was called Scott went first, followed by Mark, Dale, and me. But when we stood in line, I was the first in our family to be prayed over. Once again I felt this special sensation go through my body, but I didn't fall. Next, Father prayed over Dale. She didn't fall either. But when he came to Mark, he touched his forehead, and back he fell immediately into the arms of the usher who laid him on the floor with the rest of the "slain." Scott's turn was next, and just as quickly his eyes were closed and down he went next to his brother. Dale and I walked back to our seats as others were waiting to be prayed over. After a few minutes Mark woke up and joined us. Scott was out even longer. He then woke up and joined us, too. I asked them what it was like, but they couldn't explain it. We would definitely have to come again. I didn't know if they could be cured of their hemophilia or anything, but I wanted to keep going. The whole service made me feel closer to God.

Mark felt better when he got home and his temperature did go down to 97.4 at 7:30 P.M. But the next morning it was back up to 102.8 and he felt lousy again. His temperature continued to go up and down the rest of the week. On Thursday at 9:00 P.M. it reached 104.6. I was getting worried about him and we were going to call the doctor, but then I just had the feeling that I should give him a sponge bath with holy water. I rubbed the holy water all over him and prayed very, very hard. I think it was the hardest that I had ever prayed in my life. I begged God to heal Mark. I asked Him to give me the AIDS and take it away from Mark.

We took Mark's temperature again. It was down to 103.6. An hour later it was 102.2. I woke him during the night to give him Tylenol and check his temperature. It was 99.0. We let him sleep in the morning. He woke up at 11:15 A.M. and had a temperature of 97.0. He said he felt terrific. Was it the holy water that I had mixed from Lourdes, LaSalette, and our Lady of Knock in Ireland? I certainly felt it was.

His appetite came back and for the next three days I wrote "very good" down on his temperature chart. His highest temperature over that period was 99.3 and he was even strong enough to go for a 10-mile bike ride. Of course we didn't know that he had gone so far with his brother and a friend until they got back and the story slipped out. We thought he had done too much, but he assured us that he was fine.

The whole next week Mark was fine. He continued to do all the things he loved to do including riding his bicycle, riding his dirtbike, playing baseball, basketball, swimming, and working on his baseball cards.

Nancy Keyes came over during the week and drew his blood work. He had his gamma globulin, too. His counts were not too good, however. But he looked healthy and felt great. His only complaint was that the ankle still pained him as it did most of the summer. It was not a bleed, just the fusing of the joint that caused the pain. We continued to give him Motrin for the pain. He also complained about being very itchy from time to time.

On Saturday, July 26, Mark was sick again. But by the next day he was feeling good. The rest of the week he resumed his normal activities.

On July 31 a prayer meeting was scheduled with Father Babbitt. I asked the boys if they wanted to go and they did. My parents were also very interested, so they went up with us.

Once again, Dale and I were prayed over, but remained on our feet. Mark and Scott went out right away again. My mother did not go down either. But my father immediately fell into a deep sleep as he was placed on the floor by the usher who caught him. I was shocked that he was "slain" so easily. I was also very impressed. I would say at least 90% of the people in that church that night were "slain."

My parents were both impressed with the service and told us they definitely wanted to come back with us to another service. Mark felt very relaxed when he woke up and he didn't have the severe itching that had bothered him throughout the whole service.

July ended and I was happy that Mark had gone two months without having to be admitted to the hospital. I thanked God for this and also continued to pray for a cure. Mark had received only five vials of factor VIII all month. Two of these were for a right ankle bleed, two for a right elbow bleed, and one for a left knee bleed.

Scott was not so lucky in July. He had 13 treatments for his right ankle, a loose tooth, left knee, and right elbow.

August 1, Debbie DeMaio came for a visit. Mark was feeling great and up to his practical jokes again. Debbie was a good target because she seemed to fall for everything. Mark started her day off by slipping a false dog "mess" on the floor next to her chair. We played along with him.

"Mark, look what your dog did!" I yelled out. "I'm not going to clean it this time."

"OK," he responded, "I'll clean it up." Debbie looked down with a frown on her face when she saw it by her feet on the carpet.

As Dale and I continued to talk and distract Debbie, Mark picked up the "poops" and placed them on a paper towel. Then as Debbie watched in horror, he started to jokingly swing the towel right next to her.

"Mark!" I yelled, "Be careful with that! Go put it in the can outside."

But as soon as I finished the sentence, Debbie was screaming as the "poops" were sliding off the paper towel onto her lap. Mark started laughing hysterically and Debbie turned a few shades of deep red as she realized that Mark had got her again. Squirting pens, false money, flies in ice cubes, you name it, and Mark tried it on Debbie. And she fell for them all.

Saturday, August 2, was Mark's birthday. He was 14 years old. He woke up about 10:00 A.M. and was in a very good mood. We took his temperature and it was 98.6. Then Mark went into the family room and sat down on the couch to watch some Saturday morning wrestling. Scott walked in with a plate that had a chocolate-covered donut with one candle lit. I videotaped the action. Dale, Scott, and I sang "Happy Birthday" to Mark and then he blew out the one candle and said, "Wow, that was hard to do!"

After Mark finished the donut he said, "Now, what's for breakfast?" Dale told him he could have anything he wanted. He asked for eggs with catsup.

Then Mark started to open the cards and gifts that we had bought him. He even had a card from his dog Chipper which said, "Happy Barkday."

Dave Souza was the first visitor that morning. He came while Mark was opening his presents. Dave had white cream all over his face and neck because he had picked up poison ivy. We all made fun of him and I took close-up pictures of him.

Dale played the "Happy Birthday Mark" record that she purchased years ago. Mark loved listening to it every year. The last words were: "Happy Birthday Mark, see you next year."

Dave told Mark that he would give him a thousand dollars if he could guess what he brought him. Mark tried and tried to guess without success. So he finally gave up and opened Dave's present. It was a miniature aquarium that included a gift certificate to send away for a tadpole. Then you could watch the tadpole grow into a frog. It was called "Gro-a-Frog." Mark liked it. He asked Dave, "How did you expect me to guess that?"

"I didn't," answered Dave, "that's why I offered you the money."

"You're a big tease!" said Mark. We sent away for the tadpole that afternoon.

Mark went back to opening his presents from us. We got him a lot of baseball cards. Then Mark let out a big laugh. Dale had bought him a "Fart-whistle." He loved a good joke and proceeded to blow it over and over. He laughed and laughed, which made us so happy. That's what we wanted most for him; we wanted him just to be able to enjoy himself.

Mark also received some pictures for his bedroom, plastic pages for his cards, large looseleaf baseball card holders, a fly-shooter, buttons for his collection, clothes, a collection of small games for when he was sick, headbands, a Matchbox case for his cars, and money. When Dale asked him what his favorite gift was that we had given him, he said the baseball cards and Roger Clemens' shirt.

While Dave mixed a pitcher of Bloody Marys for the adults, Mark started using his fly-shooter. It was a plastic pistol with a string attached to a plastic circle that could be fired at a fly. It was supposed to be more accurate than a fly swatter. We didn't have any flies in the house at that time, but Mark enjoyed shooting it anyway.

Mark put a headband around his forehead and started to talk about how he would spend his money. He mentioned buying a parrot—just what we needed—another animal in the house!

Linda Nahas was Mark's next visitor. She brought her three children and her niece. We sat out on the deck. Mark was still using his crutches and had his ankle in an aircast. They gave Mark a New England Patriots shirt. Ryan and Jason went swimming in the pool. Jennifer and Becky talked with Mark and Scott. I taped everybody. Then the kids played bumper pool on the patio.

Nana Fazzina, Tony, and Sue came down next. Everyone sat around and talked. I gave Mark his Motrin for the ankle pain. He started to get itchy right away. He was miserable again. He even tried a hair dryer to stop the itching sensation. At least I figured it out, it must have been the Motrin that was causing an allergic reaction. This would be the last day of suffering because of itchiness.

Everyone had cake, ice cream, and soda. Mark lay on the glider, he was too itchy to enjoy it. A few hours later he was feeling better again. We didn't have a party for him for the first time in his life. He didn't want one because he said he was too old for parties.

Nana and Papa Hoyle also came over and Uncle Jeff. Different relatives and friends came all day long. Nana had bought him a lot of baseball cards in packages. As he opened the packs he said, "I hope I get a Dwight Gooden." One minute later he was shouting, "I got him, look, it's Dwight Gooden!"

I said, "If you get two, want to give me one?"

"Maybe," said Mark.

Chipper came over to Mark and started licking him. The dog was getting as big as a pony. "Look how nice this dog is. You're my baby, my precious baby," he said as he pet Chipper. Meanwhile, Papa was beating Scott in a game of bumper pool. But Mark later beat Papa for the championship.

Mark was tired, he had a healthy birthday except for the itching. He thanked us once again for all his presents, said his prayers, and went to bed.

The next day we all went to my sister's house to help put up a pool. We had been working on the foundation for a few days and now the site was ready. I had been in charge of leveling the ground. Mark was feeling excellent again and had a normal temperature. He helped hold up the sides while we fastened them together. He enjoyed going to his aunt's house. In fact, he loved to visit all his cousins. Ken and Nancy had two boys, Steve and Craig. Jayne and Dale had two girls and a boy, Kerry, Kathy, and Matthew. Jeff and Anne had two boys, Joshua and Adam. Jon and Carol also had two boys, Jason and Justin. So there were plenty of cousins with whom to play. Mark loved to go to family gatherings.

My parents had been thinking about moving. Once or twice a week all summer we would all spend the afternoon helping my mother clean the attic, cellar, garage, etc. Dale and I were able to do this since we were both out of work. Of course, I was getting paid by St. John's all summer. The boys enjoyed going to both grandmothers' houses and they always brought their appetites with them. As soon as Mark walked in the door he would ask, "What do you have good to eat?"

Mark and Scott went to Horseneck Beach on Tuesday. My mother went with Dale and the boys. I stayed home because I had a lot of yardwork to catch up on. My mother later told me that she saw some teenage girls looking and making fun of Mark's legs as he passed them on the way to the beach. She didn't think Mark saw them, but she did and it made her feel very bad. Mark did have thin legs, but I always told him that it was better to be thin than overweight. He never complained about his body. He was getting taller and putting on some weight and we all thought he looked wonderful.

On Wednesday, August 6, Dr. Smith met us at the high school along with Nancy Keyes and Debbie DeMaio. He had set up a 9 o'clock appointment with Mr. David Jardin, the Case High School principal, Mr. Devine (who had been appointed assistant superintendent of schools), and Mrs. Claire Howard, R.N., the school nurse. Dr. Smith just wanted to make sure that everyone understood Mark's condition at his new school. He also told them that he felt Mark should only go to school until noon. By taking away gym and study halls, it would be possible for Mark to take all his required courses, plus the visual design course which his art teacher, Mrs. Norma Currier, had recommended for him. Over the summer she had been transferred to the high school and she felt Mark had a great deal of talent in art. Mark liked her very much.

The meeting went well and then we all took a tour of the school led by Mr. Jardin. Mark thought the school was huge and was afraid that he wouldn't be able to find his way to class. Mrs. Howard told Mark that she would give him a key to the elevator to make it easier for him since he would be on crutches. She told him he could take one friend along if he wanted, but the rest of the student body was not allowed on the elevator.

Nancy Keyes came back to our house to draw blood for Mark's annual clinic visit scheduled for the following week. He also had his gamma globulin treatment. He felt terrific and even decided to lift weights on his new bench that he bought with some birthday money. Dale and I were pleased with Mark's progress. The ankle was his major problem.

Mark's latest blood results were a little better than July's. His hemoglobin was up from 7.0 to 8.1 and his HCT was up from 21.8 to 25.5. His polys rose from 30 to 64. His lymphs and monos went down a bit, but his platelets rose. His red blood count went from 3.14 to 3.51. His white blood count stayed the same, a very low 1.1 (1100). But Mark felt strong and healthy and lifted weights again.

On Friday, August 8, Dave Souza invited the whole family to go down to Newport, Rhode Island. Mark had a temperature of 98.8 and said he felt "fantastic."

We stopped at gift shops on the way down and then walked

all over the Brick Market section of the city. Mark was still on crutches, but we walked slowly, and he had no trouble keeping up with us. He didn't feel tired at all. It was a cloudy day, and there were a few periods of brief showers, but everyone had a great time. The boys enjoyed looking at all the boats in the harbor. They picked out Newport shirts and we ate at Salas' restaurant. Mark had a fabulous appetite and ate all his New England clam boil. Scott had his usual favorite, baked stuffed shrimp. The boys also played games at the arcade.

Later we drove along the scenic Ocean Drive and then passed the famous Newport mansions. We stopped at various beaches in Middletown and Portsmouth on our way home. Since it was a cloudy, showery day, we had them all to ourselves. The boys enjoyed walking along the sand and the magnificent, breathtaking views of the water.

The next day Mark went dirtbike riding with Marc Medeiros. They spent hours riding through the fields and woods. Later that Saturday Mark asked me if he could mow the lawn. It was the first time that I saw him put his foot down and actually put pressure on it since the day in June when he felt something snap while doing therapy with Sue Gemma. It was also the first time I saw him walk without his crutches. He pushed the mower very slowly and hobbled behind it. He kept taking little breaks and making faces at me as I taped him with his camera. He did five or six rows, but he didn't really have the energy for it and had to quit.

On Sunday, August 10, we went to another healing service in North Attleboro. This time, besides my parents, my brother Jeff and his family went along. They too were very impressed with the service, especially Anne who never expected to be "slain."

This was the 15th day in a row that Mark's temperature did not reach 100.0. We were so happy that he was feeling so great.

On Monday Mark went dirtbike riding again. On Tuesday it was our annual hemophilia clinic for the boys. Here are the results of that visit:

Dr. Smith: "Mark continues to do very well. His current multi-drug treatment is causing no problems. We will change his Trilasate to Feldene to see if this relieves the ankle pain.

Mark will enter high school in a few weeks. Mark should continue as is and return to see me in a month."

Dr. Melvin Hanzel, D.M.D.: "Mark does not have any evidence of tooth decay, but some gum inflammation is present. Mark also has some primary teeth present, which is unusual. I recommend X-rays to see why. He should see his own dentist fairly soon for cleaning, X-rays, and evaluation of baby teeth. An infection of the gum could occur, and this could be serious in view of his decreased immunity."

Dr. Brett Godbout (orthopedics): "Mark's main problem remains the right ankle, which remains stiff and painful with weight bearing. He is being followed by Dr. Lucas who feels the ankle is fusing. X-rays show some degenerative changes. We will try a canvas support and Feldene. If he continues to have pain despite this support, we will fit him for an AFO or some other type of rigid support. We will see him at the end of September if the ankle is not more comfortable."

Debra DeMaio, A.C.S.W.: "Mark is a bright and sensitive young man who has repeatedly demonstrated skills in expressing himself openly to health care providers, and in advocating for himself in an assertive manner. Mark and his family have persevered under a great deal of stress and uncertainty by relying on mutual caring and support, faith and humor. Continued contact planned with Mark and family."

Scott's clinic report was good. Dr. Smith talked about his anemia and left knee problems. Scott didn't have any cavities either.

Debbie DeMaio had this to say about Scott: "Scott is a bright, engaging, delightful young man who has weathered extremely difficult family health issues. His strengths continue to be his humor and outgoing personality, his many social relationships/ activities, and his close supportive relationship with family. Continued contact planned with Scott and family."

Mark spent the whole next day on his dirtbike. Marc Medeiros and Mark planned to go to Devil's Rock again. Scott, Dale, and I decided to walk there. We brought the video camera again and taped them riding the bikes and walking around on top. It wasn't easy for Mark to make it to the top with his bad ankle, but the new canvas support helped a great deal. Mark's new therapist, Sue Cotta, told Mark it was the same kind of support used by many basketball players with ankle problems. It was canvas and laced up like a sneaker. He wore it under his sneakers or his riding boots. Sue Gemma, our previous therapist, had left to go to Appalachia to volunteer her services to the needy. We had a small farewell party at our house before she left. We kept in touch by mail and phone. Sue had become a good family friend.

The new medication, Trilasate, seemed to help Mark. He became very active again. He played ball with me, his brother, and the neighborhood kids. Of course he couldn't run, but he could play catch, bat, pitch, and shoot baskets. When they played at the corner, someone always ran the bases for Mark. Everyone was really nice to him. From the 13th to the 17th I wrote down "very good" on his temperature charts. His highest temperature was 99.2 during that period.

On Sunday, August 17, we were invited down to Jack and Barbara Fazzina's summer cottage in Westport, Massachusetts. Jack was Tony's son. Dale's mother, Tony, and Sue also went down. Every year we would be invited there for dinner. The boys enjoyed going because the cottage was right on the Westport River and Jack had a motor boat. He always took us for a ride on the river and once in a while we'd stop at an island to explore it.

That day we also went crabbing. It was the first time the boys had ever done it. Jack showed them how and they baited the traps and threw them off the wharf. Some friends caught some crabs, but Mark and Scott didn't.

Later we had a big meal which started off with clam chowder, another of Mark's favorites. After dinner we watched the Red Sox, played "Trivial Pursuit," and took some video pictures. It was a fun day for Mark. He started using my grandfather's cane again because his ankle was feeling a little bit better each day. On the way home we went for a ride and ended up at Dartmouth Mall. Mark wanted to buy some two-toned jeans, but we couldn't find any in his size.

On Monday we spent a good portion of the day packing and preparing for our trip to New Hampshire. It was a good day to do it because it was pouring rain outside. We tried to take the boys on a vacation every year. They loved to go to New Hampshire because they loved the outdoors and there was so much to do up there.

In the past we had gone to Pennsylvania, Washington, D.C., New York, Virginia, South Carolina, Florida, Maine, Vermont, and New Hampshire. We would try to fit as many things into our vacation period as was humanly possible. Dale commented that she would just like to spend a leisurely vacation sometime where she could just lie in the sun all day. But her "three boys," as she called us, always outnumbered her. We liked to be active.

Mark took scenic video pictures of the White Mountains as we rode up Route 3 in New Hampshire. The first thing we did was to look for a motel. After checking out several from the highway, we decided to try the Beacon Motor Inn.

Next we drove down to a place called Clark's Trading Post. We watched the trained bear show and the kids enjoyed all Mr. Clark's jokes about bear feet, bear skin, really bear down on it, just bearly, bearries, and when the bear wrapped its paws around him, the "bear trap."

The show was excellent. Then we took a ride on the famous old-fashioned steam engine train. It even passed right under a covered bridge. We saw the haunted house and visited many of the shops in the little village. Then the boys had a great time on the bumper boats.

We had supper at the motel and then went out to play miniature golf. We bought ice cream and then browsed in a few more gift shops. I don't know who liked the gift shops more, Dale or the boys.

When we returned to the motel in Franconia Notch everyone wanted to use the indoor pool. After swimming, the family went in the hot tub. The boys played video games and then we all returned to our room for the night. Mark's temperature was 98.2 before going to bed.

The next morning we were up bright and early for breakfast and then headed north to see the "Old Man of the Mountain." The boys had seen it many times before, but never tired of it. It is a huge rock formation which resembles the head of a man on the top of a mountain. We passed the "Flume" but didn't stop since we had just been there a few years ago. We didn't stop at Natureland, Santa's Village, Six Gun City, or Storyland either.

We had seen them many times before. Nor did we dare stop at Cannon Mountain. The last time we had been in New Hampshire we had taken the gondola ride to the top. It was the scariest thing we had ever ridden. It was a very large car that held about 30 people and swayed on the cable as we went up. I have to admit that the view from the top was simply breath-taking.

This time we were on our way through scenic Crawford Notch to North Conway. We wanted to go to the top of Mount Cranmore via a nice easy one-passenger vehicle that didn't leave the ground. There were hundreds of cars on tracks that made their way up the mountain. Halfway up you did have to get off and walk a short distance to the next track. The second half of the ride was much steeper, but it sure beat the cable gondolas. We finally reached the summit and took many pictures with the video camera.

The view going down was great since you were facing the countryside rather than the mountain itself. I had the camera rolling practically all the way down.

Next we shopped around North Conway at the many gift shops there. We had lunch and stopped at a baseball card shop where the boys spent a lot of time and money. Then we traveled over the Kangamagus Highway, said to be one of the most scenic roads in North America. There are no gas stations or restaurants. In fact, there is no civilization on the entire road. But there are plenty of places where you can pull over to look at the scenery, hike, swim in a mountain stream, or picnic.

The entrance to the road is surrounded by a forest of magnificent white birches. The road then follows a mountain river as it winds its way through the White Mountains. It travels through valleys and over the tops of some mountains, and every curve brings a new marvel into view.

The boys wanted to go to Lost River Reservation. We had been there years ago and they remembered all the caves that could be explored. We thought it might be too much walking for Mark, but he insisted he'd be fine. He decided to take one crutch instead of his cane.

It was beautiful! They had all new wooden walkways that made their way along the edge of this majestic gorge. The only problem was that there were a million stairs. We were walking down the stairs, so it wasn't too bad for Mark. It had many caves to explore and Mark and Scott went in all of them.

Mark seemed to have more energy than Dale. Every time she saw a bench, she sat down to rest. She claimed she was listening to the pre-recorded taped messages. Some of the caves were pretty dark and scary according to the boys. Dale usually took the path around the caves and since I had the video camera, I only went in the ones that I could go through without crawling on all fours.

The place was loaded with waterfalls and spectacular rock formations and foliage. The clear river water actually had fish swimming in it. Mark and Scott loved the place as I'm sure every boy who went there did. Scott was a big help to his brother. He would give him his hand whenever needed and helped carry the crutch when Mark was climbing up a ladder or stairs.

The boys didn't want to stop to rest. Finally, we got to the very bottom of the gorge and looked at the stairs going up the other side. Mark almost died when he saw them. But he climbed the stairs much easier than Dale. She was all out of breath and couldn't keep up with us. Looking back at the tape later, I was sorry I hadn't offered to carry Mark on my back. But I'm sure he wouldn't have let me.

When we finally arrived back at the top there was a gift shop and snack bar. We all needed a cold drink. I told Mark that he would have no problem walking along the halls of Case High School after this workout. We bought some gifts, toured the museum, and headed back for our motel.

When we reached the motel, Mark wanted to walk around the grounds. I couldn't believe that he still had the energy to walk. We found another gift shop and, of course, Mark wanted to go in. So I went with Mark while Dale went with Scott to one of the two outdoor pools. They also had a putting green and a giant outdoor checker board with giant checkers.

When Mark saw his mother and Scott in the pool, he decided to go, too. I stayed out to shoot pictures. Mark did handstands for the camera. We wouldn't let Mark go over his head because we didn't feel that, with his bad ankle, he could swim as well as usual.

Mark had fun, but soon became cold, and like the good

brother he was, Scott got out first, got Mark's towel and brought it to the edge of the pool for him. I walked back to the room with Mark while Dale and Scott decided to try the other outdoor pool. She said it was much colder than the one they had just been in, but they both dove in anyway. Dale clowned around on the diving board for the camera. Mark changed his clothes and straightened out his new souvenirs.

On Thursday we left the Beacon and headed to Lake Winnipesaukee. We had stayed a few times at Proctor's Cabins & Motel right on the water before, and we wanted to see if they had any vacancy. They did, so we unpacked all our things and went down to the beach. It was a good-looking sandy beach and they had a large wooden deck with all sorts of chairs and loungers at the water's edge. The kids loved the beach and the outdoor ping pong table that they remembered from previous visits.

We walked down to a little shop where we bought some rafts and then floated around on the water all day. We also played ping pong and took pictures. The boys fed the ducks.

We had spent many enjoyable times on this beach in the past and the memories of the boys when they were little came back to me. We had rented rowboats and gone all over the lake. This time we decided to let Dale relax like she wanted to, so we just lounged around.

Mark went way out to the middle of the lake which scared me. I was afraid he'd fall off and not be able to swim with the bad ankle. He had always been a strong swimmer in the past, but this frozen ankle was a different situation. I finally got his attention and he came back closer to shore. He was so daring! His first question when he came back was, "Dad, what's the score?" I had been listening to the Red Sox.

At night we went down to the center of Weirs Beach. We had pizza for supper on a deck overlooking the lake. We played miniature golf and then stopped at every gift shop and every arcade.

Mark was very tired at the end of the day. We didn't know if he was overdoing it, so we decided we'd spend just one more day in New Hampshire and then head home. Mark woke up at 4:30 A.M. and complained about being cold. He had a 100.8 temperature. We gave him Tylenol and he went back to sleep until 9:30 when his temperature was 98.4. He felt much better and was looking forward to another fun-filled day.

We cooked breakfast in the cabin since we had a stove and refrigerator. The boys fed the ducks again and played one last game of ping pong. We then went back to Weirs Beach for more souvenirs and arcade games.

Next it was on to the waterslide. Usually the two boys could enjoy it. But today, only Scott could. We didn't want to take any chance that Mark would bang his ankle on the way down. So the three of us sat at a picnic table and watched Scott.

The boys wanted to drive the go-carts and we weren't too enthusiastic about the idea. But they had so much fun that they said that it was the best part of the whole trip. Later, we drove all around the lake and then headed home. We arrived late in the day. Mark's temperature was 100.4. He hadn't felt very well in the car and he took a nap.

During the night Mark woke up at 3:30 A.M. He had another one of his terrible nightmares that seemed to be coming much more frequently. He always was being chased by monsters or animals that wanted to kill him. I took his temperature and it was 98.2, which relieved me. However, the next morning it was back up to 101.6 and I wondered if Mark was going to start with another infection. But as the day went on, he felt better and went down to the corner to play with the kids. A girl named Stephanie who was in the seventh grade liked Mark and they started to "go out with each other," as they call it. They never actually go any place, but it lets others know that they are boyfriend and girlfriend.

That night Carol and Mary from Father Babbitt's prayer group came down to visit. Father had been wondering how Mark was doing and they just decided on their own to see. They both thought Mark looked much more healthy than he had the last time they had seen him.

On Sunday, August 24, Mark woke up with a headache and felt dizzy. He also complained about being sick to his stomach. This was at 6:00 A.M. His temperature was 103.0.

This was great, we complained. School would be starting Tuesday and Mark was going to be sick. He had a pretty good summer, but why was this happening to him now? I prayed to God that he would recover soon and that this was not the start of another serious infection.

Mark went back to sleep after taking some Tylenol. He didn't wake up again until 11:00 A.M. His temperature was now down to 99.2, but he said he felt weak. He stretched out on the couch in the living room, but later moved to the family room to his familiar spot. After having some toast, he took a nap. At 3:00 P.M. he was awake again and his temperature was down to 98.8. He felt a little better. But as the day went on, his temperature went up again to 100.0. But by 8:00 P.M. it was back down to 98.4. Dale and I wondered if we should even bother to take it. It was always so inconsistent. It was like a roller coaster ride. The chart that I kept was one long series of ups and downs with only a few periods of straightaways. Before Mark went to bed I asked him if I should put a "poor" down on his chart for the day. He said, "No. Put a 'fair.'"

Monday was very similar. He felt a little better, but his temperature was higher. Once again he called it a "fair" day. Before Mark went to sleep we gave him some factor VIII. Sometimes nervousness or stress can cause a spontaneous bleed in a hemophiliac. We knew Mark was very apprehensive about the first day of school, especially since he wasn't feeling his best. It was high school, it would be totally different for him than the junior high with the people who accepted him so readily. He would have new teachers, new schedules, new classes, and new classmates. He wondered how the much bigger upperclassmen would react to him. But for tomorrow, all he had to worry about were the freshmen. They would be the only class in school the first day and Mark knew most of them.

The big day arrived. It was Tuesday, August 26, my mother's birthday. The sky was bright and sunny and it was very warm. Mark wanted to get up at 6 o'clock. His temperature was 99.0. Scott also got up early. He would be starting junior high school. It would be all new and exciting for him as well. Little did any of us know then that exactly two months from that day Mark would die.

9

"Scott, if I die,
you can have all my baseball cards."

—Mark Hoyle

After a shower and a good breakfast, Mark wanted to walk down to the corner so he wouldn't be late for the bus. It's hard to tell exactly at what time the bus will come on the first day. Scott was ready to go, too, although his bus wouldn't be coming for another 30 minutes or so. So Scott offered to walk down to the corner with his brother to keep him company. Mark kissed us both good-bye as was his custom. We could not even go to the store without the two boys kissing us good-bye and waving from the doorway.

I went into the backyard and climbed up in Scott's tree house which is in the back part of the yard near the stockade fence. I wanted to see with whom Mark would be waiting. I was carefully sneaky and hid myself from his view. From the tree house you could see the corner perfectly, a distance of approximately 200 yards. I often climbed up there in the summer to see who the kids were hanging out with at the corner. Mark's tree house was closer to our house and you couldn't see the corner from there. As it turned out that morning, three girls took the bus at that corner. The bus finally arrived and Mark got on. He later told me that he sat with his good buddy, Angel Negron.

When they arrived at the school they all had to walk into the auditorium to wait for an assembly. Schedules were passed out. Mark was still limping and using the cane. He must have stuck out like a sore thumb. How many high school students do you see walking slowly with a cane?

Mark liked his schedule because it would be the same every day. He had French first period, followed by algebra, English,

217

science, history, and visual design. Once every six days visual design would be replaced by career education.

The first day went well and we were there at 12:15 P.M. to pick him up. My school wouldn't be starting until after Labor Day, so I planned on picking him up all week. Dale, Mark, and I went to Friendly's for lunch. Mark said he was pretty tired and decided to have a nap in the afternoon. His temperature was normal when we arrived home. He liked the school and was happy that he had taken a tour this summer because it was so large. Mark called the day "fair."

The next morning I picked up the newspaper and saw a heading under "Massachusetts News" in the *Providence Journal* which said: "A 14-year-old AIDS victim enters Case High School in Swansea with little fanfare. Page A-3."

The story told how Mark had "thrust the town into national limelight" last year when he attended Case Junior High School. The article did not give his last name, but did call him Mark and told how he had acquired the disease through an infected blood product for his hemophilia. Mark was just one of 1900 students who started school for the first day of class in Swansea. Remember, only the elementary schools, junior high, and freshmen attended that day.

Mr. Devine told the newspaper that there would be no extra measures taken for Mark. "I don't know if he's better, but he looks as well as I've seen him in a long time."

The newspaper had asked Mr. Devine how many class days Mark was forced to miss last year, but he would not give them a figure. He did tell them about Mark having a tutor for a few weeks and making up school work at home. "He had a good report card. He's very serious about his school work, and does it well," commented the assistant superintendent.

The paper also interviewed Reggie Desnoyers who had just talked to me the night before. Mark's former Little League manager told them how Mark would be going from "8 A.M. to noon" and how he would be dismissed from gym and study halls "to avoid getting too tired."

Because of the newspaper story, I decided to drive Mark to school. Mark had never talked to the press, except for Mark Patinkin, and I was afraid that other reporters might be waiting for him when he got off the bus. As it was, Mark liked getting a ride from me; it saved him from walking to the corner, and he could sleep a little later. We decided that I would drive him every day.

The *Fall River Herald-News* also had an article mentioning Mark. "Swansea students, including AIDS victim, back in school" read the headline. The article was very similar to the *Providence Journal* and had the same quotes of Mr. Devine. It also went into a short history of the happenings of the previous year involving Mark. Mr. McCarthy told the press that, "The whole issue was settled last year. That's the end of the report."

Debbie DeMaio visited in the afternoon. Mark had a nap before she came. His temperature was 99.8 and he still didn't feel that great. He was tired, which we expected, but we also didn't want him to get overtired. He hadn't received a locker yet, and so he was forced to carry all his books around with him from class to class. I also had to see Mr. Jardin, the principal of Case High School, to make a slight change in Mark's schedule. He was very nice to me, saw me right away, and handled the problem quickly.

Mark kept up with his homework, had me check all his work, hung around at the corner with his new girlfriend and the gang, and really seemed to be enjoying life.

Scott also adjusted very well to his new school. Since his brother had been almost a celebrity last year, we wondered what it would be like for Scott to follow in his footsteps. But Scott had no problems and he too continued to do well in school.

Mark was "fair" on both Thursday and Friday. He had naps when he got home both days and later went outside with the neighborhood kids. His temperature was close to normal.

But Friday night he woke up sick again and his temperature skyrocketed to 102.6. He was dizzy again and had a bad headache. He did get back to sleep, but woke up sick again around 11 o'clock.

He lay around all day, took an afternoon nap, and by 4:00 P.M. had a subnormal temperature. He felt better at night, but still called the day a "poor." He was upset because his friend Joey Oliveira had invited him to his birthday party and he couldn't go. All his friends went and he asked me why he had such rotten luck.

Sunday Mark was greatly improved and didn't even need to take a nap. He asked us if he could go to the LaSalette Fair, so we made plans to decorate my school room the next day and then go to the fair.

August was a good month as far as factor VIII was concerned. Mark only needed three vials — one was for his right side, one for his back, and one for the first day of school. Scott, on the other hand, had 14 treatments. They were for his right ankle, his fingers on the left hand, his right elbow, and left knee.

September 1 was Labor Day. Dale and the boys helped me prepare the classroom for Wednesday's opening and then we all enjoyed the fair. I met many people from Attleboro whom I knew including parents of students, students, and former students. All wanted to know how Mark was doing. It was very hot that day and the sun began to make Mark a little weak. So we brought him to the car, put the air conditioner on, and headed back to Swansea. He was fine the rest of the day and called it "good."

The first week of September brought more praise for Mr. McCarthy, who was cited as a local hero in the September issue of *New England Monthly*. The editors said that his response "calmed a community and set a national example."

Tuesday, Wednesday, and Thursday were "fair" days for Mark. He went to school every day, took a nap, did his homework, and then hung around with the kids. Thursday was also a gamma globulin day and Nancy Keyes was at our house to draw blood. For the third consecutive month Mark's white blood count was 1.1 (1100), but his hemoglobin went up to 8.6. His other counts were about the same with a slight increase or decrease, but nothing drastic.

Meanwhile, I was back in school. Ellen Riley and Paula Shea were new teachers at my school who also became good friends. They both were very interested in Mark and were very encouraging to me. The whole faculty was very supportive. Everyone prayed daily for Mark. Sister Martha also asked the principals to have their schools continue to pray for Mark this new school year. With that many prayers going up to heaven for my son, I had to feel very positive.

Friday was finally a "good day" again for Mark. His temperature went as low as 96.8 the previous night and stayed well below normal all day on Friday.

Once I was back in school, Dale borrowed her mother's car to pick Mark up each day and she would take him out to eat at Friendly's or Kent's for lunch. He loved the chowder at Kent's and the clam cakes. After lunch Mark would take a nap and then start his homework. That's where I would find Mark when I came home from school. He would be sitting at the dining room table with his books scattered about. He had his own desk in his room, but liked to do his homework in the dining room with the afternoon sun shining in.

On days when he felt well, he might go for a spin on his bicycle. His ankle never bothered him when he pedaled. Or he might ride his dirtbike until supper. He continued to exercise on his weight bench and talk to Stephanie on the phone.

Mark found high school very different from the junior high. In junior high the same group of classmates moved from room to room for different classes. At the high school, everyone split up after a class. You very seldom had the same people with you. You might also have upper classmen in some of your classes. Mark, being on the shy side, would have preferred to be able to walk with his friends from class to class. But he made out fine, except for the fact that the students did not get their locker assignments for a few weeks and he had to lug all his books around with him. He used the elevator, sometimes alone, and sometimes he took a friend along. Mark often talked about a girl who was in a few of his classes and who always waited for him and would hold the door for him. She was someone he had just met and he told me her name, but I have forgotten it. Yet I want her to know, if she reads this book, that Mark really appreciated her kindness.

Mark liked all his new teachers. One turned out to be Mr. McCarthy's daughter, Joanne Furze. Mark had her for English and French. Mrs. Norma Currier, the visual design teacher, would often walk with Mark to the car and help him carry the supplies he would need to work with at home. She told Dale that Mark did very well in art class last year and that he had a great deal of potential. Mark worked on some visual design signs, a sneaker, a boot, some bowls of fruit, shapes, and various other projects during September. He took his time on the drawings he made at home and showed a great deal of interest.

September 6 was a good day for Mark, but on the 7th he felt sick again. His temperature reached 101.2. He took a nap in the afternoon and by nighttime his temperature was back to normal.

He felt well enough to go to school the next day and for the next 19 days I wrote down "good" or "very good." His temperature stayed around normal and he told me that he felt "wonderful."

Life was very normal that September. Mark really enjoyed the month. He played catch with me and ball with his friends. He was even able to play a little touch football, although he had to be the quarterback because he couldn't run out for a pass. He wrote more letters asking for autographs. He sent away for baseball cards and we continued to go to card shows, card shops, and flea markets. He spent many hours reading his baseball card magazines, but also kept up with his schoolwork. He built a replica of the Parthenon for a history assignment and did a report on it, but he never had the chance to hand it in.

On the 17th he saw Dr. Smith. His blood counts were slightly improved but there weren't any significant changes. Dr. Smith was happy that the new medications for pain seemed to be working better and the canvas brace was giving Mark the support he needed.

Jody Bolton and Stephanie Ouellette (not Mark's girlfriend) were two of Scott's classmates who came over quite often to play whiffle ball and bumper pool with Mark and Scott. Mark pitched and batted. When it was his turn he hit the ball hard just about every time. I think he impressed his friends with his athletic ability even though he still couldn't walk perfectly.

Mark and Scott also liked to play "Atari." We spoiled them and bought every new tape. It was a good game for them because so often they were hurt with a sore ankle or knee and had to stay in. It kept them occupied while their friends were all out having a good time. We had over 50 tapes. Baseball was Mark's favorite. He would play that against his brother, his friends, and when there was no one around, the computer. He could beat everyone very easily.

On Saturday, September 20, the boys went on a long bike

ride. They rode down to Ocean Grove. Later they visited my sister in Touisset and fed the ducks which gathered near the Coles River. They traveled into Rhode Island and stopped at my sister-in-law's store for ice cream and soda. Nancy and Ken had bought the convenience store in 1985 as an investment and called it "Gardiner's." Mark loved to work there and Nancy had said he could any time he wanted to. He caught on very quickly and learned how to work the cash register the very first time he tried in the fall of 1985. Scott also put in some hours at the register.

We knew the boys were going for a ride, but we didn't know how far. When they came home, they had my niece Kerry with them and her girlfriend Kerr. They asked if they could give the girls a ride on the dirtbike. I told them it was all right with me, but to go slow and have the girls wear a helmet. They had fun.

After such a busy day I had expected that Mark would be tired the next day. But he wasn't; he didn't even take a nap for the second day in a row.

On Monday Mark was back in school for his 19th consecutive day. I was very pleased with the way things were looking up. Dale and I were starting our Christmas shopping early. Mark had asked for a Nintendo video game and we had bought one, wrapped it, and put it in the attic. We planned on giving the gift to both boys at Christmas because we knew they both would like it.

The rest of the week was excellent, too. I would give Mark a ride to school in the morning and Dale would pick him up at noon. He took a nap every day but Thursday. Debbie De-Maio came on Friday and thought Mark looked wonderful.

On Saturday morning he played baseball and football. In the afternoon we went shopping at Ann & Hope and Paperama in Seekonk, Massachusetts. Mark and Scott picked out their Halloween wigs. Mark chose green hair and Scott picked red. They were very expensive wigs, but the hair did look realistic, like that a rock star would have. I picked out a monk's costume complete with robe, hood, rope sash, and mask. It was a custom for all the teachers and students to dress up for Halloween at my school.

At night we were invited to a tent meeting with the Donnellys. It was a healing service by a Protestant minister. It was cold in the tent and Mark was chilly, so I gave him my jacket. The minister prayed over Mark at the end of the service and told him that he was healed. I guess the minister was mistaken.

On Sunday, September 28, Mark woke up with a 99.8 temperature and said he didn't feel well. But by late morning he was feeling much better and went for another bike ride. He still had the energy when he came home to do 10 chin-ups on the bar we had in the kitchen doorway. Mark had set a record for chin-ups this summer when he did 19 in a row. Many people tried to beat him, but most had trouble getting past six.

Later in the day Mark wanted to give Stephanie, his girlfriend, and Melissa, her friend, a ride on his dirtbike. They had fun riding around in the fields. Scott went along, too.

At night my friend Leon Cudworth and his wife Emalie came over. Usually they brought their two children, Lisa and Leon. Lisa was Mark's age and Leon was a year younger. But that night they came by themselves.

I took some video pictures of Mark and the Cudworths. He looked so healthy in them. He kept smiling and hamming it up for the camera. It would be the last time that *I* ever filmed Mark. After our company left, Mark took a shower and went to bed. He said he felt good.

The next morning Mark woke up with a 100.4 temperature and told us that he didn't think that he could go to school. He felt really bad. He had made it 23 straight days, but we definitely didn't want him to go if he wasn't well enough, so he went back to bed.

As the day went on he felt better. By 3:00 P.M. his temperature was 98.8 and by 8:00 P.M. it was subnormal. He told us that he thought he'd be able to go to school the next day.

The next morning his temperature was still low at 98.8 and he said he felt well enough to go to school. After school he took his nap and then played whiffle ball in the front yard. Then he rode his bike down to get his friend Chris Burke, whom everyone called "Burkey." But when he returned home, we noticed that Mark seemed out of breath. We asked him why he was breathing so heavily and he said that he'd been doing it for a while lately. We asked him why he didn't tell us and he responded, "I didn't want you to worry about me."

I got on the phone right away with my sister at Charlton Memorial Hospital to see if she knew if Dr. Mucciardi was in the hospital or office that week. She said he was in the hospital and she would tell him about Mark. She called back and said that Dr. Mucciardi didn't think it was anything too serious, but to come in for a gallium lung scan to be on the safe side. He scheduled us for the next day to have the dye injected and the pictures would be taken on Friday.

The happy month of September was ending on a sour note for Mark. It had been so good that he had only needed two treatments of factor VIII all month. He received them for a bleed in the groin area. Scott, on the other hand, had seven vials of treatment in September. They were for a bruise near his left eye, his right elbow, his left knee, and his big toe on the left foot.

I was very nervous about Mark's breathing. I was angry that we hadn't noticed it sooner. I remembered only too well what Dr. Mucciardi had told me back in June of 1985, "I think we can take care of this opportunistic infection this time, but if he gets another one like it, it could be a different situation." I started to pray even harder than I had been, and I prayed very hard to begin with.

Dale took Mark in on October 1 to be injected with the gallium. He said that he didn't need me to go so I went to school that day. After the injection, Dale went to my mother's house. Mark stayed there while Dale went to CVS to buy candy for her church fair. His temperature was 99.4 that afternoon and even though he said he was OK, you could tell that his breathing was not the same. Mark had me go to school to get his homework and he worked on it at night.

On Thursday, Nancy Keyes came to give Mark his gamma globulin. She also gave him his factor VIII because she was told by Dr. Smith to give Mark his flu shot and pneumonia shot. He had both of these the year before and had no problem with them. But when I got home from school it bothered me that Mark was given the pneumonia shot at this time. To me, it seemed like putting pneumonia into him when there was a good chance that he might already have it. But Dale questioned Nancy about it, and obviously she felt that it might help Mark, rather than make him worse. Anyway, there was nothing I could do about it now, it was already in his system.

Mark was still in a good mood that day and didn't seem worried about his breathing at all. Dale taped Mark in his room with his camera. He had put his wig on, a fake earring on, a large gold chain, and was all dressed up like a rock star. This is what he said on his camera:

"Hi there. I'm Mark Hoyle, the great. I have my new earring on and gold chain. Who's the coolest mama in the world? Do I look OK? I'm the coolest. Yes, I am. Yes, I am. I'm cool! Want to get a close-up of my pure green hair? Yeah! Yeah! How about a close-up of my earring? Yeah! I'm cool. Yeah, baby, I'm a cool dude!"

Mark then did a dance around his room as he made his own guitar music with his mouth. Then he continued:

"Who's the best mama in the world? Mark Hoyle. Who's the toughest mama in the world? You're looking at him, baby, you're looking at him. Yes, sir, you're looking at *him*!"

He made his customary thumbs up sign and then said, "Who's the best? Who's the cockiest? Who's the prettiest? Who's the sexiest? Who's the happiest? Yeah, you're looking at him. Yeah, yeah, you're looking at him. Yes, I'm the one. I'm the one."

He lifted his arms high above his head and faced the wall. One arm was perfectly straight, the other bent because of all the many bleeds he had into the right elbow joint. And then he said, "I'm the best. Don't listen to anyone else, 'cause I'm the best. I'm going to make a lot of money this way, 'cause I'm a punk rocker."

He then imitated playing the guitar while making guitar sounds with his mouth again. After a while, Dale cut the picture. It would be the last piece of tape with Mark on it. Looking back at it now, I'm only glad that one of the comments he made was, "Who's the happiest? Yeah, you're looking at him." That is a quote that I will never forget for the rest of my life.

Mark's temperature was 100.0 when I got home from school. I talked to him about the next day. I told him that Dr. Mucciardi would meet us at the hospital to look at the X-rays and then advise us on what to do next. There was a chance that he would hospitalize him. Mark told me that he thought that was what would happen. I reminded Mark that Debbie DeMaio was coming next week, and he had to stay healthy because he had promised to show her how well he rode his dirtbike.

Dale thought that Mark would definitely be going in again, too. She started to get pajamas and other items ready. I reminded them both about how sick Mark was when he had breathing problems last year. He had high temperatures, he couldn't eat, he couldn't even walk because he was so weak. This time I felt we were catching the problem much earlier and everything would be all right.

Then Mark shocked all of us when he came out with this statement: "Scott, if I die, you can have all my baseball cards."

"Mark," I said, "what are you talking like that for? I've never heard you talk like that before, where's your positive thinking? A winner never quits and a quitter never wins! It's never too late to rally!"

"I don't know, Dad," he said, "I just don't know."

Was Mark a lot sicker than we thought? Did he know something that we didn't know? I blocked it out of my mind and gave Mark another pep talk. And I did feel positive. Everyone was praying for Mark. God wouldn't let me down. "Ask and you shall receive" I kept thinking. God would take care of Mark. He would cure him. He had to. We were too close and I couldn't live without him. God knew how I felt about Mark. He had to make him healthy again. He had to!

Mark woke up at 5:00 A.M. Friday morning, October 3. He felt sick and his temperature was 102.0. I gave him Tylenol and he went back to sleep. He slept most of the morning since the gallium scan was not scheduled until the early afternoon.

When we went to Charlton Memorial Hospital, Mark walked in. He underwent the tests and then waited for Dr. Mucciardi to come down to look at the X-rays. My mother came to the hospital and sat with us. My sister let us wait in her office.

Dr. Mucciardi came, looked at the X-rays and then had us go into a room and look at them, too. They showed definite changes from the pictures that were taken earlier this summer. He said that Mark should go into the hospital for another bronchoscopy to see what was going on.

He gave Mark his choice of going to St. Anne's where he would do the bronchoscopy, or going to Rhode Island Hospital where he had been so much lately and where he might feel more comfortable.

"What should I do, Dad?" Mark asked me.

"I think that you should go to St. Anne's and have Dr. Mucciardi do the bronchoscopy like last year. Then if you want to be transferred to Rhode Island Hospital, that could be arranged."

"Yeah, I think that's the best idea, Dad. Why don't we do that?" Mark responded.

We left the X-ray department and went to our car. We had everything ready for a hospital visit. Mark even had us bring his school books so he could keep up with his work. I drove directly to St. Anne's.

I went to the desk to fill out the papers while Dale went to the gift shop with Mark. He looked at stuffed animals because, even though he was a teenager, he still liked them when he was in the hospital. But he decided to get baseball cards instead. He also bought five pieces of bubble gum. It's funny how some things stick out in your mind.

We ended up in the same room as last year. It had been done over, but basically everything was the same. Dale went out to get a pizza because that's what Mark requested.

Nana Fazzina was waiting for Scott when he got off the bus and she brought him to her house for supper.

Besides eating the pepperoni and mushroom pizza, Mark also had a tuna fish sandwich. Dale bought him a new robe, new pajamas, and new bear feet slippers. Mark loved the slippers. They were about a foot long and had brown hair all over them and toes like a real bear's foot.

Nana and Papa Hoyle came up Friday night with Halloween treats and decorations for his room. He had an IV started. Dale decided that she would sleep there and I would go home with Scott.

Mark told his mother that she "was being less nervous than Dad this trip to the hospital. Usually it was the other way around."

They didn't give Mark any oxygen, but he did ask to have his fan blowing toward him so he could get more air. He had a very peaceful night.

When Mark woke up the next morning, Saturday, October 4, he was sick. He walked into the bathroom and vomited. Later Dale told me that "like a nut, I was concerned because he threw up on his new slippers."

I arrived very early after leaving Scott at Nana Fazzina's. I brought the factor VIII that Dr. Mucciardi asked me to bring for the bronchoscopy. I mixed it and then gave it to him through one of the IV needles so I didn't have to stick him.

Mark asked us to go over during the operation to the store that he could see from his window. He wanted us to buy some strawberry soda.

We walked Mark to the operating room for the sixth time. We kissed him good-bye and wished him good luck. It was just as difficult to leave him as it was the very first time.

Dale and I went to get a cup of coffee, and then we walked to the store to get him the soda that he wanted.

Scott had volunteered to work at the church fair that day. Mark had planned on working there, too. He had made the candy airplanes the week before.

Mark came back from the operating room and said, "It wasn't that bad." He was still groggy and wanted to know if it was over. He was tired and he fell back to sleep.

Dale left to go to the baseball card shop for him. He had wanted some complete sets that he had ordered a while ago for "a real bargain price." The man had Mark's name in his folder for ordering certain items. The man told Dale, "Boy, your son sure got himself a good deal here. He knew exactly what to buy, and what was a bargain!" She returned to the hospital and Mark was happy to see all the cards when he woke up.

Relatives and friends came to visit Mark during the day. He spent the rest of the day resting and breathing more easily because they gave him an oxygen mask.

At night my parents were there along with Dale and me, and Mark said, "Dad, I think it would be better if I just died. Then you wouldn't have to worry about me anymore. And then I could watch over you."

"Mark," I said, "please don't talk like that. We love you very much and I don't mind worrying about you at all."

My mother also commented to Mark, "Mark, we all love you. Of course we worry about you. But we'd rather have you here to worry about." My mother later told me that a funny feeling passed through her when Mark said that.

These negative comments were so unlike Mark that it scared

me. Why was Mark talking like this? I looked at Dale, she looked at me, but we couldn't say anything more. It hurt us both so deeply.

I stayed at the hospital that night while Dale slept at home with Scott. Mark had a very restless night and a touch of diarrhea. I had to keep getting him the bedpan, and he wanted the fan blowing on him, too. I didn't mind doing anything he asked me to do. I felt so bad for him. It just didn't seem fair that he had to suffer so much. He should have been home in his own bed. He should have been going to school with his friends and enjoying life. He should have been playing sports and going out with girls. He shouldn't have had hemophilia either. Why Mark? Why Scott? What did they ever do to deserve such a fate? I was very depressed, but I couldn't let Mark sense it. I had to be strong for him, as always.

The cold air blowing on him from the fan made me nervous. I did not think it would help his breathing, but hinder it. But I asked the nurse and she said it wouldn't hurt him. I felt better.

Dale came up very early Sunday morning and Mark had more visitors as the day went on. Betty Neilan, my godmother, once again sent me a check to help with gas money. She had been the best godmother a person could have.

On Sunday, Mark's breathing seemed to get worse as the day went on. He was still in a pretty good mood, though, and talked to us all day. He was given oxygen. He still had the diarrhea during the day, but he was not nauseous. He slept a lot.

At night I went home with Scott and Dale stayed at the hospital. Mark was given a blood transfusion. The doctor had a difficult time finding a vein and wanted to use Mark's foot. Dale would not let him. She told him that Mark and his father had been putting needles into his veins for years and they were not experts. He kept trying and found a vein in his arm. Last year at St. Anne's he had a nurse stay by his side during the whole transfusion. This time, they left him alone, short of help I guess.

Mark had a miserable night, his breathing was difficult, he still had the touch of diarrhea and he was extremely restless.

I arrived early and was shocked by his condition. He had been 100% better the night before when he kissed me and hugged me and told me how much he loved me. Now he seemed to be struggling for breath. I asked Dale if the nurses had seen him and she said yes. I immediately went right to the nurses' station and begged them to give him more oxygen. All he had was the kind with the two little tubes that went up his nose and the setting was real low. She called a doctor, he ordered a blood gas. The results showed what I knew all along, Mark needed more oxygen. A bigger face mask type with more oxygen seemed to give him some relief.

Mark was still very uncomfortable. Dr. Mucciardi came and told us outside Mark's room that he needed more care than St. Anne's could give to him. He ordered an ambulance. Mark would be transferred to Rhode Island Hospital. Dr. Mucciardi also told us that Mark was a very sick boy this time. We asked him how he could be so sick so fast. He even walked into the hospital this time, just Friday afternoon. That's how pneumonia hits you, he told us, it just all of a sudden blossoms out. Preliminary tests seemed to point to pseudomonas. Dr. Mucciardi told us that they would probably ask us at Rhode Island Hospital if we wanted to put Mark on life-support systems. We said that we certainly wanted to do everything possible to help Mark.

I felt terrible! Mark was really suffering! I felt so helpless. I hated this damn AIDS virus that was so microscopic and yet had caused such a large problem in this world! In *our* world! I prayed that the doctors at Rhode Island Hospital would find a cure for this latest strain of pneumonia.

My mother had come up to the hospital early, too. She knew that Mark's condition had really worsened and wanted to be there to do anything she could for any of us.

We told Mark that he was going to be transferred to Providence. He said, "Can you ask the ambulance driver to put the siren on all the way there? I like the siren." We promised that we would.

They gave him pain medication and it seemed to make Mark very sleepy. I guess it was to make him more comfortable for the trip. He wanted me to go in the ambulance this time. He remembered that his mom had gone the last time.

As he was being wheeled out of the room, he asked his mother this question, "Could you stop at Paperama on the way to the hospital and get me a squirting pen and fake ice cream sundae

that I saw there a few weeks ago? I want to play some jokes on
the nurses."

Those would be the last words that we ever heard Mark speak.
All the way up in the ambulance he had his eyes closed and
never talked. I was getting sick to my stomach and was so
happy when I finally could step out of the ambulance. I could
imagine how sick Mark felt. My brother Jon was there to greet
us when we arrived. He worked in East Providence at the time
and my mother had called to tell him how sick Mark was. Besides the medical technician, a very nice nurse came along
with us and stayed with Mark until he was taken care of in the
children's intensive care unit. It turned out that her sister had
just moved to our street.

A tall woman doctor met us in the emergency room and
walked with us as Mark was wheeled through the maze of corridors to the I.C.U. I was allowed to go right in with Mark. All
the doctors and nurses immediately went to work on him.
They asked me to leave for a few minutes and then they put
Mark on a respirator. I don't even know if they knocked him
out or what, but when they let me back in, Mark was sleeping
peacefully with a large tube stuck down his mouth into his
lungs. I had to answer the usual questions. Dale hadn't arrived
yet. My mother and Dale had stopped at Paperama to get the
jokes that Mark requested. But soon Dale was at my side again.
The date was Monday, October 6, and up to that point in my
life, it was the worst day I had ever experienced.

The only thing that gave me some comfort was the fact that
Mark was not struggling for air anymore. The machine pumped
the required amount of oxygen into his lungs. Now, if they
could only cure this pneumonia he had, we could fix him up
and take him home, I thought.

I asked the nurses a million questions. I wanted to know
what all the machines were doing and what the numbers meant.
This was my son they were working on, and I had to find out
everything I could about the care they planned for him.

The nurses told me that they hoped when Mark woke up,
he wouldn't try to fight the machines. If he could just let the
machines work for him, it would be a lot easier for him. Otherwise, they would have to knock him out with this medication
called pavulon. I prayed that Mark would not try to fight it. But

I had a feeling he would. I understood how difficult it would be not to fight it. You want to breathe on your own, at the rate you're used to, you don't want a machine breathing for you. But I wanted Mark to be able to communicate with us. If he didn't try to fight it, he would be able to stay awake. He wouldn't be able to talk because the tube passed right over the larynx, but we would know how he was because he would be able to write down things and shake his head to our questions. I prayed and prayed that he wouldn't wake up and fight it.

He started to stir, I knew he was waking, I was there to tell him to relax. But he panicked! He tried to pull the tube out of his throat. The nurses had to hold him down. I begged him to be calm, but he kept trying to fight the machine. They had to give him the pavulon.

I was so disappointed. Now we wouldn't know how he felt at all. I bet he was scared stiff. I held his hand, and Dale and I talked to him as if he was awake. We explained where he was, why he had the breathing tube, and how the doctors and nurses were working on him to make him better.

All the time, he lay perfectly still. The pavulon, I learned later, is a drug that completely paralyzes the body. The pygmies of Africa used the drug in their blow guns to hunt animals. It would freeze you completely so you couldn't move a muscle. The animals would die. So would humans if they weren't on respirators. The respirators did the breathing for you and kept you alive.

The problem was that since Mark was now on the pavulon, we wouldn't know when he was awake and when he was asleep. We talked and talked to him, but did he hear us? He might be sleeping and not hear a thing. We decided it would be best to repeat things a lot at different intervals during the day. That way there was more of a chance that he was awake and heard us. But if he was awake, how did he feel? His eyes were closed, he couldn't even blink. Was he thirsty? Was he hungry, sick, in pain, or scared? We didn't know. Did he have an itchy leg, nose, or arm? If he did, no one would know. He could be awake, want to move, and be so frustrated because he couldn't move or talk. It had to be one of the worst experiences a person could have! I felt terrible. I kept imagining how I would feel if I was Mark—frozen in a state of limbo. Over and over we tried to explain what was happening and why he had to stay like that. The doctors and nurses told us that patients on pavulon can hear clearly. They know what is being said to them. But the doctors are not sure when they are awake or when they are sleeping. Patients who are very sick do a great deal of sleeping.

Mark also had a catheter put up his penis and they put some tubes into some veins near his heart to monitor it. It was terrible to see all this equipment.

I had never heard of a respiratory therapist, but I soon learned all about them. They were in charge of the respirators and also cleaning the tubes which had to be done quite often. At first, they made us leave the room because it wasn't pleasant to watch, but as the days went on, we were allowed to stay. I could see why they had made us leave. It was a torturous procedure for the patient. They would unhook the tube at a mouthpiece and then squeeze some liquid down into Mark's lungs. You could see the scared expression on his face even though he couldn't move. Then they would give him a little more air and then stick a narrow tube down the larger tube and suction liquid up. The liquid was from his lungs. You could see how frightening it would be to Mark. They would have to cut off his oxygen while they suctioned. It must have seemed like he was going to suffocate. Oh, poor Markey, I felt so bad for him!

I told him over and over that we loved him and not to get depressed and give up. He had to keep fighting. He had to get better. We were counting on him. We understood how frightened he must be. But we would not leave him alone. I squeezed his hand, I brushed his hair, I rubbed his face, I kissed him, I even opened his eyelids so he could see me once in a while. I didn't know if he was awake or asleep, but we talked and talked and talked all day. I kept telling him that they gave him medication so he couldn't move. It was not permanent, I told him over and over.

This is what the nurse wrote in his record that first day:

Temp. 101, Pulse 168, respir. 82, B.P. 138/84, 11:00 a.m., 10/6/86. Mark is a known hemophiliac who has AIDS. He was admitted to Pediatric Intensive Care Unit as a transfer from St. Anne's Hospital due to deteriorating respiratory status and worsening respiratory distress. On admission to P.I.C.U. Mark is awake and responsive but acts drowsy. He is aware of his surroundings and is anxious if his parents are not with him. He is in 100% Oxygen but is cyonotic with dusky nailbeds and mucous membranes. His skin is warm and dry with good pulses and fair perfusion. He is nasal flaring with supra clavicular retracting and using abdominal excessory muscles, his breath sounds are equal bilaterally and very coarse with a minimal wheeze in his LLL. He was medicated and then intubated with a #7 cuffed ET tube and put on the respirator. His breath sounds remained unchanged and his color became pink with only slightly dusky mucous membranes. He was suctioned for moderate amounts of loose, tanish-orange secretions. Once he woke up and began assisting he resumed his nasal flaring and use of excessory muscles to breathe and began popping off the vent. He was medicated with morphine without effect, then valium without lasting effect, and finally pavulon with good effect. He was placed on the cardiac monitor in a sinus tachycardia. During his entubation he became bradycardic. He had an arterial line inserted by Dr. Weissman with a normal arterial tracing which drew back easily. He had an IV in his left antecubital infusing. He had a NG tube inserted and placed to gravity drainage. He had not voided and no bladder was felt but he had a foley inserted and drained amber urine. Debbie DeMaio was called and spent the afternoon with the parents. Problem: alteration in respiratory status related to impaired gas exchange and ineffective breathing pattern.

D. Travers, R.N.

Debbie Levesque, R.N., was Mark's first nurse and she was very helpful in answering our many questions about the things that Mark was going through. Debbie DeMaio was also a tremendous help to us, not only that first day, but every day that we were there. Nancy Keyes, R.N., also visited us every single day. The hospital chaplain, Father Malino, came by often to talk to us. Dale's minister, the Rev. Dr. Tavitian, came to comfort us as well as Father Jim from St. John's. Father Jim administered the Sacrament of the Sick to Mark.

Dale was extremely upset that first day and could not sit in with Mark for too long. It hurt her too much. I tried to stay strong for all of us. I continued to talk positively and I really felt that way.

My father left work to come to the hospital. Dale's parents had to wait for Scott to get home on the bus and then they came up with him. Scott went in to see his brother. He didn't stay long because he felt so bad for Mark. He never wanted to go back into the P.I.C.U. again. He cried for his brother for the first time.

All our relatives came up to see Mark. The room across the hall was a parents' lounge and my family practically filled it. Only two could be in to visit Mark at a time and the hospital rules said immediate family only. But our relatives had been so supportive to Mark throughout every illness that the nurses let them in as long as only two were with Mark at a time.

Dr. Smith was not very hopeful at all. He told us that Mark was an extremely sick boy and probably wouldn't make it past Wednesday. I didn't believe a word of it, but Dale did.

My brother Jon and I spent the most time with Mark that first day with other relatives coming in to relieve Jon. I didn't want to leave Mark's side when he needed me most. But Jon talked me into getting some sleep around 1 A.M. and I agreed. He said he would stay with Mark until around 3 A.M. and then wake me. He also promised to wake me right away if anything serious developed. I slept on a couch in the parents' room across the hall. Dale and Scott were already sleeping there when I walked in. Mark had an uneventful night.

In the morning Scott wanted to go to school. So Dale drove him home about 6 A.M. After showers and a change of clothes, Dale brought him to school and then went home again to gather some items for the hospital. She brought up some pillows, some food, toothbrushes, razors, clothes, etc.

Dale was better able to tolerate Mark's appearance on Tuesday. It did take a lot to get used to seeing all the tubes and machines. They tried turning Mark on his side, but he didn't endure the move well and had to be returned to his back. His peep, which was the amount of pressure being pumped into his lungs, was set at 9. The day before when he came in it was set at 8.

The doctors talked to us about getting a kinetic bed for Mark.

They thought it would really help his lungs to have him constantly moving.

Mark was still on pavulon. Before a new dose was given, Mark would come out of it a bit. We would ask him questions and ask him to respond by squeezing our hand. He did this with no problem. I guess the hands are the first parts to get movement. It felt great to know that he could hear what we were saying to him. It was almost like he was in a coma while under the pavulon.

One of the nurses told us about her sister who was on a respirator with pavulon for months. She eventually recovered from her illness and later talked about how the family had talked to her. She remembered a good portion of what they had said to her. The nurse encouraged us to read to Mark and keep talking to him. So we did. I read the newspaper to him, particularly giving special time to the sports pages. I read the get well cards he received to him over and over to be sure that he knew that all his friends, classmates, and relatives cared about him.

Peter Fontaine, R.N., was a big help to our family. He was a very understanding young man who had a lot of compassion and was an excellent nurse. He understood what we were going through and always took the time to explain everything he was doing. I'm sure Mark liked him very much. Peter talked to him all day, too. When it came time for Mark's daily sponge bath, Peter would let me stay inside the drawn curtains. I would help Peter take the bed apart so we could wash Mark. It felt great to be able to hold his head in my arms. Usually his head was held in by the cushions and you could see just his face.

Peter's girlfriend, Patty, was a secretary in the P.I.C.U. She was very friendly, too. In fact, they both were good friends with our next door neighbors, Rita and Kelly Brennan.

The kinetic bed arrived on October 8. The nurses had described it to us and it really was something to see. It was metal with green pads all over the top that stood out about 10–12 inches. There were green pads on each side of Mark's head and green pads under each arm. Pads ran down his sides and between his legs. There were pads for his feet and three heavy straps like seat belt straps to hold him in place. Once he was all strapped in, they would set the bed in motion. It would slowly turn on its side until Mark was completely sideways. Then it would start up again and turn toward the opposite side. Mark must have been very frightened although we all tried to reassure him that he wouldn't fall out. I was nervous that the tubes would get tangled and unhook from his mouthpiece. And it did happen a few times!

Mrs. Linda Shea, R.N., was the representative from the kinetic bed company. She had attended Sacred Heart Academy in Fall River with my sister although she was two years older. Jayne had even dated her brother Bob LaFlamme. It was such a small world.

Mrs. Shea told my sister and us how successful the bed had been. It had worked with everyone who had been put on it. Of course, Mark was the first AIDS patient to use it.

The nurses were instructed to continually inform Mark about what was going on, even if they were just holding his hand. The doctors told them to explain to Mark why he couldn't move and to frequently reassure him that he was not going to fall off the kinetic bed.

On October 9, Debbie DeMaio had this to say in the charts: "Parents coping styles quite different from each other. Father still confident that Mark will recover fully; mother seems to be beginning the anticipatory grieving process. 11-year-old brother has been with parents in evening and overnight — has opted to attend school every day. I am trying to get some time with Scott to allow him some opportunity to express feelings, fears, etc. Parents have expressed strong wish to shelter/protect brother from the fear/sadness of Mark's critical medical status. Extended family, community, and school supporters continue to visit Mark and family. Father persuaded a 'healing priest' who has prayed over Mark in the past to visit last evening, which reinforced father's stated belief that Mark will live."

Father Babbitt did come to Rhode Island Hospital along with Carol and Mary from the prayer group. They all prayed over Mark and then Father Babbitt prayed over him alone. He gave me a Padre Pio relic and told me to hold it on Mark and pray over him often, at least once a day. I did as he suggested, many, many times a day. Father Babbitt told me when he was leaving that, "It is in God's hands."

Since I was at the hospital 24 hours a day, the whole time

seems almost like one big blur to me. I do know that Mark had many visitors. I'm sure I would leave some out if I tried to name them all, but I would like to name the people who were there most often: Billy Brodeur (Mark's friend—he knew he couldn't actually go in and see Mark, but he came up just to see us and ask how he was doing.), Mary Patricia Medeiros, Nancy Harkness, Dave Souza, Maureen Bushell, Robin Sherman, Linda Nahas, Sue Travers, Sharon Marchand, Father Jim, Mr. Devine, the Donnellys on returning from a Florida trip (they came right from the airport when they called home and learned Mark was in the hospital), Sister Martha, Father Smith, Mary Braga, Franny Powers, Louise Dunphy, Jeannine Vignali, Carol Hilsman, and Rev. Dr. Tavitian.

Superintendent McCarthy also came up with Mr. Jardin. Mr. McCarthy was so shook up after seeing Mark that he had to leave the room. Mark did look pitiful. Besides rotating on his bed, and having tubes coming out of his mouth, nose, heart, arms, etc., he had white gauze pads over his eyes because of an eye infection he had contracted.

One day Bishop Cronin of the Fall River Diocese came up to see Mark, along with Monsignor Oliveira and Father Hessian. I was very impressed with their kindness in coming all that way to see Mark. It was a day I will never forget. With the bishop praying for my son, he had to get better, I thought.

Our family really helped us by staying up all night with Mark while we got some much needed sleep. Since we had promised him that he would never be left alone, we wanted to keep our bargain. Dale and I tried to spend part of the night with him, but it got too much for us. So, as we slept on the couches across the hall, Jon, Ken, Jayne, Nancy, Dale Wilson, the two Nanas, and my dad took turns staying with Mark.

The hospital eventually gave us a room at Gerry House which is where the residents stay. It had a shower and a place to hang our clothes. We kept extra food there and all our toiletries. We never did spend the night there, choosing instead to sleep on the couches in the lounge across from the P.I.C.U., but it was great to have the room. Dale did take some afternoon naps there and every morning when Dale's mom and Tony arrived, we would go there to shower and change.

Susan Bartulevicius, R.N., didn't have Mark as a patient, but was very nice to us all. She was a very understanding nurse who really cared about her patients. Claire Piette, R.N., was another very sweet nurse whom my family all liked. Most of the nurses were super; there were only a few who seemed to have no compassion at all.

On Thursday, October 9, Mark remained in critical condition. But to me, it was great that he had hung tough. I had remembered what Dr. Smith had said about Wednesday. The doctors weren't sure that he only had pseudomonas which had shown up on the cultures taken at St. Anne's by Dr. Mucciardi. They thought he might have Legionnaires' Disease, or pneumocystis, or M.A.I. (mycobacterium avium intracellularus), or cytomegalovirus. All these affected the lungs. He was given tests for all of them and given antibiotics to cover. He was also again put on some experimental drugs, of which we readily approved.

Dr. Smith suggested using a nose trach. It would be easier for Mark, he thought, if the tube went up his nose and down his throat. We were all for anything that would make it easier on Mark. They did it that day. Mark certainly looked much more comfortable with that large tube up his nose instead of in his mouth. The other nostril had the small tube leading to his stomach.

On October 10, the residents decided to wean Mark off the pavulon. We weren't too excited about this because we knew how he had fought the machine the last time and we didn't think he was really ready for it. It was good to be able to ask him questions though, as he lightened up a little. He could nod his head a bit and squeeze my hand on command, but he was very scared.

I asked him if he wanted me to buy a dirtbike when he got better so I could go riding with him. He squeezed my hand to signal yes. I asked him if he wanted us to extend his room to make it bigger. He squeezed my hand to signal yes. I asked him to squeeze my hand if he was in any pain. He didn't squeeze. (Later during his stay he did signal that he was in pain.) I asked him to squeeze my hand if he was afraid. He squeezed my hand the hardest he had done all night. He hated the bed, wanted me to wet his lips, and was very uncomfortable. All this I learned through hand squeezes. As the pavulon continued to wear off, he got more and more agitated and fought the respirator. His head started to bang into the pads and he began to move his feet around. He didn't want to answer any more questions and you could see how worked up he was getting. I hated to see him suffering, but that's what was happening. He was trying to breathe against the machine and it kept popping off. His blood pressure was rising and so was his heart rate. Some of the nurses began to tell me that I should ask the doctor to stop the experiment. I did ask him if he could give Mark more pavulon because I felt the present treatment wasn't working. Mark just wasn't ready yet. One of the nurses was really getting upset and suggested to me that I should call Dr. Smith about this. I hadn't thought about that, but I decided it was a good idea and left to use the pay phone in the hall. Dr. Smith listened to me and then hung up and called the unit. Soon they put Mark back on the pavulon.

The nurses all were relieved and so were we. Mark rested comfortably for the rest of the night with the respirator doing the breathing for him.

Not much happened on the weekend. Mark's condition remained critical. Jayne took Scott shopping for some new clothes to wear on his class trip that was coming up that week. He was going to the Boston Museum of Science by bus. Dale had told Jayne to get Scott whatever he wanted.

Mark's eyes were checked by an expert and the drops she gave him made them less red. At least he didn't have an infection in his eyes anymore, which was some good news. He did have a bloody nose one morning. It was probably due to the tube rubbing against his nostril when the bed rotated. I continued to ask all the nurses a bunch of questions. A couple of them thought that I was testing their knowledge, which wasn't the case at all. We had always played such an important role in Mark's medical care and I just wanted to know everything I could about the machines, what the numbers meant on the monitors, and the medications he was being given.

Each day when it was almost time for Mark's pavulon, we did get to ask him questions and he responded. We were always happy to know that he wasn't in any pain, but we were saddened by his fears. Of course, we understood that fear, a fear that even an adult would find very difficult to live with, much less a 14-year-old boy.

On Columbus Day, Monday, October 13, the nursing staff had a meeting with us about visiting status. They asked that visitors be limited in order to allow Mark to get more rest. This was a contradiction to what most of the doctors had been telling us. They had told us to talk to him all the time. If he was sleeping, he wouldn't hear us anyway, but if he was awake, he would be happy to hear our voices. Some of the nurses disagreed with the other nurses over this issue. One even told us the story of one teenage girl who was on a respirator on pavulon and the father kept telling her that he would buy her a new blue car when she recovered. She was on for over a month before she was strong enough to come off the respirator. Her first words were, "I want a white one." She was talking about the color of the car.

We disagreed with the staff and made our feelings known. We felt that Mark needed the full measure of support from all his family to recover from this infection. We had always been a close family and Mark always had loved company. I showed the staff some magazine articles that supported our belief.

Some improvements were made on the 14th. Mark was able to move his mouth, nod his head, and squeeze hands in response to questions when the pavulon was wearing off.

On the 15th, some edema was noted in Mark's ankle and upper arms. It was decided that a therapist should come and work on Mark's arms and legs every day.

Our family had taken over one of the closets in the lounge. We had all kinds of soda, cups, cupcakes, cookies, chips, etc., stored there as well as magazines, newspapers, and items for Scott to amuse himself with at night.

There was a color television there and the Red Sox were in the play-offs, which everyone watched. Since Mark had watched games with me all spring and summer, I would put the Red Sox games on for him in the P.I.C.U. He couldn't watch them, of course, but he could listen. I explained all the action to him and sat with him for all the games and the World Series, which also began while he was in the hospital. We hung Red Sox banners on his wall and everything. One nurse wanted to shut the game off because she said it was getting Mark too excited and his blood pressure was going up. This got me really angry, especially after Dr. Smith had said the day before that Mark could have the games on. She said that she didn't care what Dr. Smith said. I knew that Dr. Smith said that he wasn't concerned about the pressure during the game. And I was happy that it did go up. It showed that he was listening to the game.

The whole time that Mark was in the hospital was an emotional roller coaster for my family. There were so many ups and downs on Mark's vital signs and respiratory readings. His peep had to be raised all the way to 16 at one point. We were all on edge and not getting our proper rest. Scott continued to spend every night at the hospital with us. He never went back into the P.I.C.U., however. Dale drove him to school every morning. He went every day, kept up with his work, and made the honor roll.

When Mark was at St. Anne's hospital he had asked Nana Fazzina to find a good home for Chipper. Mark loved the dog, but he was getting too big and too hard to handle. So Dale's mother asked around. Meanwhile, she continued to go down to our house every day to feed Chipper and the cats. Since Chipper was left alone so much, he started to destroy things. He wrecked our patio door, our kitchen sliding screen door, and all our outside chair cushions. The foam was scattered all over the yard. Nana found a nice home for Chipper with a family who had just lost a German shepherd. They loved Chipper right away and we were all happy that the dog would get more attention than we could give him at this time. We never told Mark about this, even though it was his idea.

Meanwhile, cards and letters continued to pour in from relatives, friends, and classmates. And I continued to read all of them to Mark over and over, especially the ones from his girlfriend Stephanie.

Scott went on his class trip to Boston and Mary Patricia Medeiros picked him up along with her daughter Lisa when they returned. Scott ate supper at Lisa's house and then Mary Patricia brought him up to the hospital. He brought souvenirs back from Boston for Mark, Dale, and me.

The next couple of days were uneventful, but on the 20th X-rays showed a gradual improvement in the lungs. Tests also showed an improvement in pulmonary function. It was hard to pinpoint an attributable reason because of so many variables, but Dr. Smith and Dr. Erica Jost, an infectious disease specialist, were both thrilled about this. They brought us into a room to show us the X-rays.

I told Mark all about it, over and over. "Your lungs are getting better, Mark," I said. "I knew you could do it. The X-rays are showing signs of improvement. Keep fighting!"

But I was also concerned about his general health. He had not eaten since October 5. I knew he was getting IV feedings, but I wondered if they were enough. With so many medications going into his system, I thought they would wreck his stomach. They had tried to put food down his tube a few times, but Mark had not tolerated it well, yet I thought they should try again. I also worried about his feelings. Was his throat dry? Was his mouth dry? I'm sure he was very uncomfortable but couldn't tell us his concerns.

Dr. Smith wrote in the chart that "we should probably be able to stop the paralysis once the respirator setting is lower." Was he starting to get positive, too?

Debbie DeMaio took Scott to the Swansea Mall so she could talk to him alone. But Scott would not discuss his brother. He did, however, respond to the individualized attention she gave him.

By the 22nd, Mark's peep was down to 6. He was really making progress from the 16 he was at the week before. Things looked much brighter for Mark and I continued to feel very positive. I kept telling Dale that everything would be all right. God would take care of Mark. Mark was special, he had hundreds of people praying for him. God wouldn't let all these people down.

Sue Cotta, our therapist, continued to exercise Mark's limbs. The problem was that fluid was building up in his arms, legs, and feet. He also had bed sores, with a particularly bad one on his left elbow. But his peep was down to 5 on the 23rd.

On the 24th Debbie DeMaio wrote: "Parents somewhat less anxious today feeling Mark is doing better in some respects. 2½ weeks of less sleep, eating disruption, as well as total life disruption is wearing on parents. Mark's extended family and friends continue to show great support. Both the Catholic Church and Protestant Church also show much support."

Both my mother and mother-in-law had psychic experiences that reinforced my faith while Mark was in the hospital. My mother was at home saying her daily novena and thinking about Mark. It was after midnight and she was sitting in her favorite chair in the den. While she was praying, she suddenly felt as though someone was blowing in her ear. It startled her, and she turned quickly to see if someone was there. But no one was there. It happened again. It scared my mother, but she took it to mean that God had heard her prayers for Mark.

Dale's mother also had an experience. She was lying in bed worrying about Mark when she heard a voice say, "Don't worry, he'll be all right." It was a woman's voice, but she didn't recognize it as one she knew. Both these signs made us feel better.

Irene Fournier, a friend of my mother's, also had an unusual experience. She dreamed that she saw the Blessed Virgin Mary standing with her arm around a teenage boy. She had never met Mark, but she felt the boy in the dream was Mark. He looked so happy and content, she said. She interpreted the dream to mean that Mark would get well again because Mary was protecting him. Later, after Mark had died, she attended his wake. She was astounded when she looked at Mark because he was definitely the boy in her dream.

On Friday night, I had a terrible dream; I dreamed that Mark had died! It was almost quarter of 4 in the morning and it woke me up in fright. I got up off the couch, put my shoes on, and hurried to Mark's bedside. Dale's mother was spending the night with him and all was peaceful. I didn't tell her why I had gotten up. "Just checking on him," I said, and then I kissed him and went back to the lounge. But I couldn't get back to sleep.

On Saturday morning, everything seemed OK, and Linda Nahas talked Dale into leaving the hospital to get a haircut. She really needed to get out; she had been living at the hospital in Providence for 20 days!

But the good morning turned sour. Mark's blood pressure went up and his fluid status was increasing. The respiratory therapists had to increase the peep again. It was a major setback.

Dale returned with a new shorter hairstyle and looked terrific. She felt good until she learned of Mark's setback. Then she had to leave his bedside because she felt ill. I continued to be positive, to me it was just a minor setback. Scott went home with Linda Nahas. He was asked to spend the night with his friend Ryan. It was the only night that he did not spend with us.

Dr. Barudi, covering for Dr. Smith who was away, told me about another setback. I can't really remember what he told me, but it was something about Mark's blood cells eating other cells. It sounded horrible!

The rest of the day Mark continued to get worse. All our company left and it was just my mother, Dale, and me. I was planning to divide the night with my mom while Dale slept.

The nurses told me that the doctors wanted to put a new catheter into his heart because they needed more information with this new setback. They had pulled the other one a day or so before when it had failed. I didn't want them to do this because Mark seemed like he was in such a weakened condition.

Each time they suctioned him, he had a very difficult time. I wished that they could just leave him alone. My mother tried to get some sleep while Dale stayed up with me. His readings, which I could understand by now, were extremely poor.

The doctors arrived to put the catheter in after midnight on October 26. We left the room and waited patiently until they were finished. By 1:15 A.M. they were done and we went back to Mark's bedside. The machines continued to give out poor readings and the peep continued to be raised. I was totally depressed and so was Dale.

It was time to suction Mark again. He had struggled each time that evening and I wished they didn't have to do it, but they did. As the nurse suctioned him, the machines started to nosedive. Mark's blood pressure was going down, down, down before our very eyes! It was as low as 30s/20s! Mark went into cardiac arrest! The nurses and doctors rushed to his bed. They coded him and Dale and I left the room. We couldn't take it any longer! Our Mark was dying!

Dale was crying. My mother came out of the lounge and started crying, too, when she heard the horrifying news. I stood there with my wife hugging me on one side, and my mother on the other side. I just couldn't believe it! Why, God? Why?

Dr. Barudi arrived and went right into the P.I.C.U. He came back out to inform us of Mark's extremely grave condition. I was physically and emotionally exhausted. I turned pale and began trembling. I couldn't control myself, I was shaking all over. Dale and my mother brought me into the lounge and had me lie down. One got a nurse while the other got me some wet paper towels. I could not describe the terrible feelings that I had inside of me if I tried. I just felt like I was falling apart! The nurse brought me some Valium tablets and water. I took them and they must have worked, because I eventually stopped shaking.

I felt very hurt, mad, and embarrassed. Hurt, because Mark was dying, mad because God had let me down, and embarrassed because I was the man and I was supposed to be strong. But instead, when it came right down to the end, Dale turned out to be the strongest. She and my mother had to take care of me!

The nurse came in to tell us that they had gotten Mark's heart going again. She asked us if we wanted to go back in with him. I couldn't go! I just couldn't! I couldn't stand to see him die. I knew that he would and that the dream I had was going to come true. I looked at my watch. It was 3:35 A.M., at quarter of 4 the night before I had awakened with the nightmare.

Debbie DeMaio had been called and was with us in the lounge. My mother stayed with me while Debbie went in with Dale. The chart said that "Mark continued to deteriorate despite all the measures taken."

Dale held Mark's hand and was with him during his final moments. He died at exactly 3:44 A.M., October 26, 1986. I felt so terrible that I couldn't be with him at the end, but I thought he would understand. On October 26, just two years prior, Mark had gone to his very first dance at the junior high.

Dale came into the lounge to tell me the crushing news. We hugged each other for the longest time. I felt incredibly sick. An empty feeling passed all through me. The nurse gave me some more Valium.

Dr. Barudi came in to comfort us. Then he talked to us about an autopsy. Would we want one performed? I said that I would if it would help other AIDS victims. I wanted to know exactly what it was that took our son's life.

My mother called the relatives to give them the sad news.

My niece Kerry Wilson was having a slumber party at my parents' house. All the girls knew Mark and cried very hard. My father, two brothers, and sister all came up to comfort Dale and me. I was still in a state of shock as I sat on the couch in the lounge. Dale had Jayne and Debbie go with her to Gerry House to get our belongings. Everything from "our" closet in the lounge was brought to the cars. Then we left. Jayne drove our car for us.

We sat and talked in our house. Dale and I had a lot of "why's." Why did Mark have to die? Why did he have to suffer so much? Why did God let us down? Why did they have to put that wire into his heart? Why did they have to suction him when he was having such a difficult time? The "why's" flowed out of us, but there were no answers.

When it was a decent hour, Dale went for Scott. She decided that there was no need for both of us to go pick him up, so Dale went alone with the difficult task of bringing the sad news to Scott. It was a beautiful, sunny morning which reminded me of an Easter morning.

Dale went inside Linda's house and said to him, "Scott, I have something I have to tell you."

"What is it?" he asked. "Did Mark get worse?"

"Yes, Scott, he died last night," Dale responded.

Scott broke down and cried as Dale reached out to hold him. They hugged each other tightly as they mourned the loss of son and brother.

Dale's parents came down to our house. Family and friends gathered to console us. Father Jim came down from Attleboro. We all talked, and talked, and talked some more.

Scott asked if he could play "Paperboy." That was the large video arcade that "A Wish Come True" had given to Mark. We said yes because we thought it would be good for him to get his mind off his brother for a while. He plugged it in, but the music didn't come on as usual. Instead, for the first time ever, a message blinked across the screen: "Insert Coins. Insert Coins." Scott couldn't believe his eyes! The boys had played the game thousands of times before and this had never happened before. He called us all into Mark's bedroom to look. The machine that had been programmed to never use coins would not work. I gave Scott two quarters. He put them in the coin slot and immediately the music and machine came to life. Scott played the game and the machine went off when he was finished. Usually after playing a game all we had to do was push the button, and a new game would start. Instead, it flashed, "Insert Coins. Insert Coins." I told Scott to unplug it and try plugging it in again. The same thing happened. "Insert Coins. Insert Coins," the message read. We took it as a sign from Mark that he was OK. He loved money, and he would save and save for the things he really wanted, like baseball cards. He always worked hard for his money. This was his game, this was the day he died, it was like he was sending a sign to us.

10

"Mark taught us all a very important lesson,
one that will guide us through our lives.
He taught us to live as full a life as possible
and to make the best out of what seems to
be the worst. Mark is our hero and
we'll never forget him."

—Dedication in the
St. John Evangelist School Yearbook

D ave Souza came up with the idea of a scholarship to be
given in Mark's memory. We thought it was a great idea.
The Mark Gardiner Hoyle Memorial Scholarship Fund would
be established and we would encourage donations instead of
flowers in Mark's memory.

The first trustees were David Souza, chairman, Jeffrey Hoyle,
Marnie Lancashire (a teacher at Case Junior High School), Joanne Furze, and Kenneth Gardiner. The scholarship fund address was established as: Mark Gardiner Hoyle Memorial Scholarship Fund, c/o Swansea School Administration, 1 Gardner's
Neck Road, Swansea, Ma. 02777.

Later the committee drew up the papers and this is what
they said about Mark:

"A Scholarship Trust is created in memory of Mark
Hoyle, an extremely courageous young man who, in spite
of a long lasting and very difficult illness, demonstrated
to family, friends, teachers and to the general public that
a full and fruitful life can be lived under the most adverse
of circumstances even though the number of years available to him were few. Mark, a quiet, considerate and caring fourteen year old lived a life filled with love for his
very dedicated family and pursued many interests, hob-

bies and sports which helped him to pass his many days of illness and frequent hospitalization without complaint and with the highest degree of courage up to the time when his illness no longer would allow."

Student recipients of the scholarship would be selected by a majority vote of the trustees. They would give special attention to students who had demonstrated a good scholastic aptitude, but they didn't necessarily have to be honor students. Further considerations would be given to financial need and to the student's involvement in the athletic programs at Joseph Case High School. The recipients didn't have to be members of the athletic teams, but could be involved through lending assistance, being student managers, or being enthusiastic suggestors of school activities.

Dale and I decided that all the money put into Mark's machine "Paperboy" would be donated to the scholarship. Scott, his cousins, and friends all continue to play the game.

Funeral arrangements were made with the Waring-Ashton Funeral Home. We wanted Mark's wake to be held in Swansea, the town that he loved and called home. Rita Brennan, our next door neighbor, and Dave Souza accompanied us to the funeral home to make all the arrangements.

Both Dale's church and my church were very small. We thought it would be nice to have the funeral in a larger church and we chose Holy Name Church in Fall River because that is where Dale and I got married. Monsignor Daniel Shalloo and Rev. Dr. Leon Tavitian, who both took part in our wedding ceremony, would also be there for Mark's funeral. Monsignor would say the mass and Reverend Leon would speak. My good friend Father Jim would give the homily.

Dale's deceased relatives were all buried in Warren, Rhode Island, and my family's deceased relatives were buried in Fall River. But we wanted Mark to be buried in Swansea and chose Mt. Hope Cemetery.

We knew the wake would be very difficult so we decided to have just one day, Tuesday, October 28. The funeral was scheduled for the next morning.

Mark's classmates learned about his death from Mr. Jardin. The principal had called the whole freshman class to the audi-

torium to inform them. They had a moment of silence for
Mark. Then Mr. Jardin told the class about the scholarship in
Mark's memory.

According to Joey Oliveira, a friend of Mark's, the rest of the
day the students didn't do much work. The next class for Joey
was Mr. Mulligan's algebra class. He called the class off because "he was sad like the kids," according to Joey. "When we
went back to class after the announcement," Joey said, "I couldn't
work anyway because I was crying and couldn't concentrate on
my work. Mr. O'Hare, my guidance counselor, came into my
French class and took me down to his office because he wanted
to talk about Mark's death. He wanted to talk to me because
I was a good friend of Mark. He also talked to Marc Medeiros
and others. That day in Career Education class a lot of kids
cried."

On Monday evening, October 27, the *Providence Evening-
Bulletin* had a front page headline: "Swansea boy dies after bat-
tling AIDS—Town rallied around stricken youngster."

"Mark Gardiner Hoyle" the article started. It was the first
time Mark's full name was printed in the press. The story went
on to tell about Mark and how Swansea supported him. Mr.
McCarthy ordered all flags to fly at half-staff for Mark.

All the local TV stations had feature stories about Mark.
They interviewed Mr. McCarthy, Mr. Devine, friends, and
teachers. Here are some of the comments made on the various
channels:

Mr. McCarthy: "Anytime a child dies, it is very tragic, and
in this particular case, since we did have the opportunity to
share in Mark's life, it's particularly touching. And now it's a
time of grief for his parents, his family, and we certainly join
in that."

David Gorman (a friend): "He was a nice kid, he was a good
friend. He was always happy. I never saw him in a bad mood,
it's a shame that it had to happen to someone like him, he
really enjoyed life a lot."

Brian Geary (a friend): "The last time I saw him he was
really up. Nothing seemed to get him down very much. He was
always up."

Mr. Devine: "Mark was a very real, animated, very popular young man. He was afflicted with a deadly disease. He never lowered his head, he stood tall, he greeted all of his classmates with a smile, and they treated him the same way. I'm very proud to have been Mark's principal and also very proud to have been the principal of all of those students at Case Junior High School who contributed toward making the last year of Mark's life just about as good as it could be. One of the things that I've learned from all this is that if decent people are given the opportunity to do the right thing, they will. And I think that's what happened in Swansea. Mark was right up there on our lists of heroes. He set an example for all of us to live as full a life as possible."

Dale (speaking to Dave Layman, a local newscaster, on the telephone): "Mark truly believed that he was going to make it. He rode a dirtbike, had a girlfriend, and was accepted by his fellow students. He was in remission just before he died. In lieu of flowers, contributions may be made to the Mark Gardiner Hoyle Memorial Scholarship Fund."

Ann Conway (WLNE newscaster): "He was known only as Mark, but now the Swansea high school student who had AIDS is dead. Tonight we can tell you his name. His name was Mark Gardiner Hoyle. He was only 14 when he died over the weekend. And it was tonight that I found out all the things that Mark did to make him such a hit with his friends and his family. Mark Hoyle was a Little League All-Star, a big Red Sox fan, he drove a dirtbike, he won art contests, chess championships, he had a girlfriend, he never talked about his illness."

Brian Geary: "Nobody mentioned his illness to him, so he didn't feel any worse about it. You could talk to him. He was never down."

Ann Conway: "Mark collected pictures of celebrities and said he would have liked to go public as Ryan White, the Indiana AIDS victim, did. Mark loved being in school with his friends and became the first AIDS student in the country who was allowed to continue with school."

Mr. Jardin: "Mark blended right in. Mark had courage and I think that gave other people confidence. So much so that I always expected to hand Mark his diploma in four years. He gave you that kind of feeling that he was going to lick it, that he was going to win. That's the type of individual he was. And I think that's the thing that affected all the kids, they thought Mark was going to win."

Mrs. Currier (Mark's visual design teacher): "Mark was dedicated, mature, serious about his work." (Larry Estepa of WJAR asked her what she thought the hardest part was for him.) "Probably knowing what was to come, but he had a lot of faith and I think that really helped him get through."

Mr. Estepa: "Close friends wouldn't talk about Mark's death, or couldn't, the way you don't talk about a friend behind his back. But Mrs. Currier says, 'They'll be there tomorrow.' If you didn't know him, you'd probably say he was an innocent victim of an insidious disease. But if you did, you'd know he wasn't that at all. He was, in fact, what he always wanted to be, just another freshman at Case High School. One of his friends said, 'He always looked you right in the eye because he didn't have anything to hide.'"

Channel 12 showed pictures of our house, Channel 6 showed Mark's yearbook picture, and Channel 10 showed pictures of Mark's art work at Case. We didn't grant any live interviews with the press.

Sue Travers told the press, "I think we all had hoped that things would be different. Mark's family never ever gave up hope. He touched a lot of people and they touched him. Each time a school district would allow an AIDS-stricken child to attend classes in another part of the country, I viewed it as a victory for the Hoyles and the residents of Swansea. Because of Mark, it will be easier for other AIDS victims to attend school. He gave people a chance, and we'll never be sorry for that."

Reggie Desnoyers said, "It hit me like a rock. I knew Mark was in the hospital but I wasn't overly concerned. He frequently entered the hospital for AIDS-related complications. I wasn't banking on any miracle medicine, but I thought that being a kid, he was going to beat it. Baseball was his thing. The kid tried so hard to be better than he was."

In his obituary we mentioned that he was an honor roll student in his freshman year at Case High School, that he had been a Science Fair project winner for two years and a Principal's Award recipient while at Case Junior High School. We told how he was a former Swansea Little League All-Star pitcher and shortstop and an avid baseball card and autograph collector.

Dale talked to the *Herald-News* on the phone. She told them that: "Mark just seemed to bring out the best in people who were involved with him. He always thought he was going to make it. He was in remission all summer and felt great. He rode his dirtbike, played baseball and went to the arcade. Then he went to school where he enjoyed a visual arts course, did his homework, and tried to please us with achievement in school. He was a regular kid, he never asked for special treatment." Dale then related the story about the Halloween costume.

Dale continued, "This trip to the hospital, one of many, was not going to be different. We thought, honest to God, he would make it. He was such a fighter. He always pulled through." Dale then related the story about playing jokes on the nurses, telling his brother that he could have his baseball cards, and telling me that we would be better off if he was dead.

"But Mark was not on a pedestal," Dale said. "He could be a brat like any other 14-year-old. It was a family decision to let him lead a normal life."

Dale, Scott, and I all had prescriptions for Valium. It really helped us get through the wake. We chose a red hooded sweatshirt and dungarees for Mark with his white socks and high top sneakers. Dale also wanted some pictures of Mark to be mounted near the casket. We chose some of him riding his dirtbike, playing basketball, and clowning around in the house with his clothes stuffed like an 800-pounder. We also placed the jokes that Mark had asked us to get, his last words, near his casket.

The line at his wake was so long that visitors had to wait an hour before they could even enter the funeral home. And then the line stretched on from there all the way down the hall and right to the casket. All this support kept Dale, Scott, and me completely occupied all afternoon and evening. It truly helped us tremendously that people turned out like they did. Mass cards, spiritual bouquets, donations to the scholarship fund, flowers, and cards poured in.

Not only did we get cards and letters from our friends, but also from complete strangers. Here is an example:

Dear Mr. & Mrs. Hoyle:

After watching the disappointing World Series loss on television, and the subsequent tears in the Red Sox dugout, I went upstairs to read my evening paper. I was jolted back to the real world by the headline article involving the loss of Mark. How I thought could I have been so emotionally involved in a meaningless sporting event when people like you are going through such remorse.

I join with my family in offering you our prayers and heartfelt sympathy. Having children of my own I cannot relate to the reality of your loss. . . . It's too difficult to even imagine!

Mark must have been a very special young man to have received the love and support that was extended throughout his illness.

For whatever comfort this letter might bring, you should know that perfect strangers care, and in a different, but sincere way we weep with you.

Sincerely, John P. Bergmark (Barrington, R.I.)

Wednesday, October 29, was another sunny day. Our morning paper, on the day of Mark's funeral, had an article by Mark Patinkin. He praised Mark, Mr. McCarthy, and Swansea.

Mr. Patinkin said, "I had to keep reminding myself that Mark had AIDS. He seemed so content with his world. It must have been because he knew how much his world embraced him."

Mr. McCarthy told Mr. Patinkin that the students of Swansea took something out of all this. "They came to see that if a kid's down," he said, "you get behind him. Mark taught them that and they'll always take it with them."

I received a phone call from my former college roommate at St. Anselm's, Peter Barry. He had driven all night from his home in Pennsylvania and had just arrived at my brother's house across the street. He didn't want to disturb us because he knew we would be busy getting ready, but he offered us his condolences and told me he would see me at the services. Mark had always liked Peter and his family. Pam and their two children, Shawn and Paula, had visited us often and we spent many enjoyable days at their home as well.

We arrived early at the funeral home, but already there was another line waiting to say a prayer before Mark's casket. The waiting rooms were full of people. Many people who had not been able to make it the night before were there including many of my students from St. John's. Sister Martha closed the school down for the day. Many doctors and nurses from Fall River Pediatrics, St. Anne's Hospital, and Rhode Island Hospital were there. Many other doctors and nurses had come the night before.

The time arrived for people to be called to their cars. It took a very long time. While I was waiting, I kept wondering if Mark could see all that was happening from his new home in heaven. If he could, he must have been really impressed. How often does someone get a funeral as large as this one? And to have a school closed in your honor? How many Massachusetts funeral processions are led by Rhode Island State Police? They had called to offer their services. And Mark must have been pleased that two of his baseball favorites, cousin Greg Gagne and Russ Gibson, were at the wake as well.

Finally, it was our turn to say our final good-byes to Mark. We kissed Mark and put some of his items into the casket, including a baseball cap that the Swansea Little League had brought to the wake. Dale stayed the longest, giving Mark one last kiss.

The funeral procession left the parking lot led by the two Rhode Island State Police officers in their award-winning uniforms, followed by the Swansea police. As we pulled out onto the street, there was a Swansea police officer stopping traffic outside his patrol car. When we turned onto Route 6 east there was another Swansea patrol car blocking traffic with another officer. At the next set of lights there was a Somerset patrol car and police officer. We had three more sets of lights to go through in Somerset and at each one there was an officer who had stopped all cars for our funeral procession to pass.

I thought how proud Mark must feel. I was sure he could see everything that was happening. I looked back down Route 6 from the top of the hill in Somerset, and the cars were as far as I could see. The newspapers later said the procession was more than a mile long. They also said it was the biggest funeral procession ever in Swansea's history. "God Bless a brave young boy Mark G. Hoyle," said a sign in a local Swansea appliance store front window.

When we finally arrived in Fall River and turned into Hanover Street where Holy Name Church is located, I couldn't believe my eyes. They had the whole street blocked off for the funeral procession. I had attended many funerals there before and never had I seen this done before. Cars were then parked four across from curb to curb.

Sister Mary Jessica Aguiar, R.S.M., the former principal at St. John School in Attleboro, had volunteered to put a mass booklet together. It added so much to the service.

Dale, Scott, and I entered Holy Name Church arm in arm as the Case Junior High School Choir under the direction of Mr. James LaFlame sang "The sun'll come out tomorrow . . . better hang on till tomorrow, there'll be sun." The song was from the musical *Annie*. Mark had so enjoyed watching the performance his classmates had put on back in the spring. It was a song of hope. Mark had loved the song.

It was a long walk down to the front row pew. Gail Rey, the funeral director, led the way. She was so helpful to our family throughout all the proceedings. The church was full. I wondered if there would be room for everyone who came in the funeral procession.

The opening hymn was "On Eagle's Wings." While they wheeled the coffin to the foot of the altar everyone sang:

> *"And He will raise you up on eagle's wings*
> *Bear you on the breath of dawn*
> *Make you to shine like the sun*
> *And hold you in the palm of His hand."*

The pallbearers took their places in the front row opposite us. They were Kenneth, Stephen, and Craig Gardiner, Jeffrey and Jon Hoyle, Dale and Matthew Wilson, and Marc Medeiros.

Monsignor Daniel F. Shalloo, pastor of Holy Name Church, was the principal celebrant of the mass. He was joined by Rev. James Fitzpatrick and Rev. John Smith of St. John the Evangelist Parish. Also present on the altar was Rev. Dr. Leon Tavitian of First Christian Congregationalist Church; Rev. William Campbell and Deacon Orosz of St. Dominic's Church; Rev. William Babbitt of St. Mary's in North Attleboro; Rev. John

Cronin, of Our Lady of Fatima, Swansea; Rev. Marc Tremblay
of Notre Dame, Fall River; and Rev. Mark Hession of Holy
Name, Fall River. Father Jim had told me that Bishop Cronin
wanted to be there, but he was out of town. The altar boys were
from my eighth grade class: Michael Dolan, Brian Healy, and
Christopher Sabourin.

John E. McCarthy, Swansea superintendent of schools, read
from Lamentations 3:17–26. "My soul is deprived of peace," it
said in part, "I have forgotten what happiness is; I tell myself
my future is lost, all that I hoped for from the Lord." The Re-
sponsorial Psalm was "Be Not Afraid." The refrain is: "Be not
afraid, I go before you always. Come follow me, and I will give
you rest."

Harold G. Devine, assistant superintendent of schools, read
from 2 Corinthians 5:1, 6–10. "Indeed we know that when the
earthly tent in which we dwell is destroyed, we have a dwelling
provided us by God, a dwelling in the heavens, not made by
hands but to last forever. . . . "

After the gospel about Lazarus, John 11:17–27, Father Jim
gave the homily. Here is the complete text:

How ironic it is, really, that as we gather here this morning in sadness—in emptiness—with tears . . . we gather
for a celebration of life! Those of us here who knew Mark
Hoyle personally *know* why this funeral mass for him
must be a celebration of his life.

Normally when we think of coming to a funeral, we
think of a grandparent, or an aunt or uncle . . . someone
older, who has perhaps had the chance to live a long life,
someone who dies of old age. We can expect those things
to happen. What makes Mark's death different is not so
much that he was so young (14 years old), but that in those
14 years, he was able to do so much . . . to be so much . . .
and to enjoy so much of life in such a short time.

We all know the circumstances of Mark's sickness and
death. And something else that makes Mark's death different for us is that he was able to share it with us . . . he
never fully hid his illness from those who knew him, and
so for many who are here today . . . you were able to walk
along with Mark, and many times suffered along with
him, especially during this last illness of his.

Today we come here to Holy Name Church to celebrate his funeral: and we must ask ourselves: who was Mark Hoyle to *me*? Sure, we know that he was a son, brother, grandson, nephew, neighbor, schoolmate, friend, cousin — and fellow Christian. And in these relationships, what did Mark give us . . . what were his gifts to us?

Mark was obviously a likeable kid — outgoing to people with so many different interests: I know personally that baseball was his passion (having gone twice with his family and 8th grade from St. John the Evangelist School to the Baseball Hall of Fame in Cooperstown . . . at this point, Mark could give the tour). He was bright . . . eager to learn new things and enthusiastic about whatever he was involved in. His mind was always turning . . . wondering perhaps how he could make more money to further his baseball card collection . . . and always thinking about the future. He loved his dirtbike . . . animals . . . and he loved school. Even in spite of his many illnesses, Mark continued to maintain a place on the Honor Roll (which cost his parents big bucks when it came to report cards). Mark had even gone to school every day this year until his illness of three weeks ago.

And so what were Mark's gifts to us? All of these qualities we see in Mark Hoyle were things that he shared with us. However . . . it would make no sense at all for us to call them gifts, unless we were to take them as examples for you and me to live by.

One of Mark's gifts that must be mentioned, indeed, is his gift of faith — given by God, but given by his parents at Baptism. And certainly when we talk about gifts as being examples for others to live by . . . you're talking about Mark. For the believer in Christ, sometimes life will require things from us . . . sometimes Christ Himself will ask things of us that are very hard for us to respond to. And again . . . when we look at the gift that Jesus has been to the world, then as believers it is good to take on His example and to live by it . . . not just in the "party" moments of life, but also in the difficult moments of life, as it was for Mark.

I would venture to say that faith has also been an important part of the lives of all Mark's family and friends—after all—how often did we *all* pray for Mark at one time or another: that he would get well again . . . that a cure for his disease might be found . . . and seemingly here today, our prayers have gone unanswered.

Oftentimes our faith is the only thing we have to hang on to after someone close to us has been taken away. Christ's promise of a newer, better life "where there are no more tears . . . no more pain" sounds nice but sometimes doesn't do anything for the pain we feel inside.

In the first reading we heard from Lamentations, it sounds like the person who wrote that has perhaps experienced something similar to what we feel in losing Mark. "My soul is deprived of peace . . . I have forgotten what happiness is . . . all that I had hoped for from the Lord. . . . " But part way through the reading, the whole mood changes: and suddenly the author realizes that all is not lost, "The mercies of the Lord are not exhausted, they have not come to an end . . . they are renewed each day . . . so *great* is God's love for us!!!"

Saint Paul in the second reading also speaks about being confident and having hope during the darker moments of life's journey: but for us, now that Mark is gone, we *wonder* about that hope.

Jesus in the Gospel had some friends: Mary, Martha and Lazarus. We know that He visited them from time to time. Lazarus died one day and Jesus went out to see what He could do for them there . . . we know that Jesus felt very bad about losing *His* friend . . . *He* even cried. Martha went out to meet Jesus, and quite plainly told Him: "If you had been here sooner, my brother would never have died." How many of us here thought the same thing about Mark? If Jesus *really* heard my prayers for Mark, then would this terrible thing have happened to him? And what Jesus said to Martha, He says to each of us here today: namely, that God has not abandoned Mark. . . He never did, even during his illness. Because for Mark God's goodness is not over— now he has found that peace that no drug or medicine could give him . . . the Lord has indeed healed him. And very much like Lazarus, Jesus has called forth Mark. . . He has "untied" him from the sickness, the pain that weighed him down . . . and just like Lazarus, Jesus has "let him go free."

Oftentimes we can feel that a funeral means "the end" of things. Today's funeral for Mark is a little different, though: for those of us who were so hopeful, so confident for Mark, we might be tempted to take those dreams and hopes and bury them with Mark today—but we cannot do that because that would mean defeat—quitting—giving up . . . and that wasn't Mark at all.

"A quitter never wins . . . and a winner never quits: it's never too late to rally." Those were Mark's own words . . . he lived by them and relied on them, especially when things looked bleak.

And perhaps that would be Mark's message to us today: don't stop living because I'm not here . . . never quit hoping . . . never quit dreaming . . . look ahead, because there's always time to change things. HOW IMPORTANT THAT IS ESPECIALLY TO ALL THE YOUNG PEOPLE HERE TODAY . . . WHEN THINGS LOOK BAD FOR YOU, AND YOU THINK YOUR PROBLEMS ARE BIGGER THAN YOU ARE . . . NEVER GIVE UP HOPING THAT THINGS WILL GET BETTER, BECAUSE *MARK* NEVER DID.

Even with sad hearts, empty hearts and broken hearts, we gather as the family and friends of Mark to celebrate his life. We celebrate the Eucharist—the word itself means "thanksgiving"—and that's just what we do: we give thanks for the gift of Mark: who/what he was to us. We give thanks for the example of hope and courage that he was to all of us . . . we give thanks that the Lord enabled all of us: doctors, nurses, family, friends to help him . . . and in so doing, perhaps he made all of you the heroes.

We show our thanks in the Eucharist by offering bread and wine which will become for us the presence of Christ . . . and as we offer these gifts, may I suggest that from our hearts and minds, we offer on the altar our memories and thoughts of Mark, in thanksgiving to God for allowing him to come into our lives even if for only 14 years.

To Dale and Jay and Scott . . . very few of us know how you feel today, but know that we feel with you in your loss. In closing, I would like to read a verse that has become popular . . . it has been the theme of the "Friends of Mark" of Swansea. . . .

Footprints

There was a man who had just died and was reviewing the steps he had taken during his life. He looked down and noticed that all over the mountains and the difficult places he traveled, there was only one set of prints but over the plains and down the hills, there were two sets of prints, as if someone walked by his side.

He turned to the Lord and said, "There is something I don't understand; why is it that down the hills and over the easy places you have walked by my side, but where the places are rough and difficult, I walked alone, for in these areas there is only one set of footprints."

Jesus turned to the man and said, "It is true, that while your life was easy, I walked along by your side, but here when the walking was difficult, I realized that was the time that you needed me the most, and that is why I carried you."

No . . . we do not leave this funeral empty. Christ promises to walk with us, to help us carry the burden of this grief . . . and to give us the understanding we need to know the "why" of Mark's death.

"The sun will come out . . . tomorrow." That was Mark's song of hope yesterday . . . hope that he would get better . . . hope that there would be a cure for AIDS . . . now, the sun has come out, and that sun is the eternal light of Christ, who has come to call Mark to be with Him in the everlasting kingdom forever. Amen Alleluia!"

How inspirational . . . how moving . . . how comforting. . . . Father Jim knew just the right way to say everything. I was so pleased that I had asked him to give it. I hoped all the young people in the church would remember it.

The service continued with the "Prayer of the Faithful" read by Rev. Dr. Tavitian. He offered a prayer for Mark and "those who gave Christian witness in his last illness"—school officials, teachers, doctors and nurses at St. Anne's and Rhode Island Hospital, and the Friends of Mark volunteer support group.

David Souza, Nancy Harkness, and Maureen Bushell brought up the gifts for the Offertory. The Communion Hymn was "Let There Be Peace."

When the Case Junior High School Choir sang, "You can always count on me, I'll be at your side forever more, that's what friends are for," many students and adults broke down and wept.

The recessional hymn, played by the organist Raymond Whalen, was "Ode to Joy." Dale, Scott, and I left the pew and started down the aisle the same way that we had walked in — arm in arm. It was then that I realized how many were in the church. Newspaper accounts said that over 600 people attended.

Later, in a letter from a friend, we were told, "At the funeral mass I could see in my mind, Mark between Jesus and Mary holding hands, smiling at you, Jay, Dale, and Scott; and the understanding then came: that all of you will be taken care of." I prayed that she was right.

The TV cameras were across the street and shot footage as we walked out of the church. We quickly got into our pale yellow limousine. The pallbearers brought Mark's casket into the hearse and we left for Swansea. Once again the police were waiting for us in both Somerset and Swansea.

We passed Elizabeth Brown Elementary School. Mark had been a student there. We passed the junior high and scenic Swansea dam. We entered the cemetery and circled around to Mark's gravesite. It was a beautiful, peaceful spot. From there you could see the Brown School on the south. Directly east, just beyond the hill, you could see the top of Case Junior High School. A short distance to the north was Case High School. To the west, a few hundred yards beyond the woods, were the Little League fields where Mark used to play.

Over 300 persons gathered for the graveside prayers. Father Jim Fitzpatrick, Father Smith, and Rev. Dr. Tavitian all spoke.

When they were finished we asked for the cluster of brightly-colored balloons, which had been kept off to the side. Dale handed them to Scott and he released them into the clear blue sky of autumn. The newspapers said that "many of the mourners wept as Mark's family watched the flight of the balloons." We were facing north and the bouquet of yellow, red, green, and pink balloons were gently swept in that direction toward Case High School.

We stood and watched their flight until they were just a speck in the sky. Dale, tears in her eyes, then turned and took a flower from Mark's casket. She then took a ribbon. We went back to the waiting car.

After we left the cemetery, I was told by friends who stayed that the teenage mourners then walked to the grave and picked flowers from the mound of bouquets that covered Mark's brass casket. I guess they wanted something in remembrance of their friend.

Many cried and cried. A teacher told them not to cry for Mark because he wasn't in pain anymore. "Remember him, and live for him," the teacher said.

Edward J. Durand, news editor for the *Fall River Herald-News*, wrote this beautiful piece which deeply touched my whole family. He has given me permission to use it. The title was: "Mark drew from us the power of love: He moved us all in a quiet way."

Rest now, Mark, the journey has ended. All your trials are over, young man. There are no more mountains to climb. There are no more rivers to cross. There are no more tests of hope and courage. Your pain is gone now. The long dark night has called your name as it does to all of us. But you have gone into the dark night with a light that guides us all.

Rest now. No more will the cruel winds find you vulnerable. You are gone to another place where peace is your eternal reward. Your soul has taken flight in sweet surrender. Though you leave us here with a sense of loss, you leave with us your courage and you leave with us that overpowering sense of a love that you have generated, a love that will always return to those who knew you best and miss you most.

What is more tragic than the death of a young person — with all the dreams that will never be fulfilled and all the laughter now but a memory. Those who knew him saw in him the joy of living, even as his health failed. If fate seemed to call all too early and all too cruelly, Mark did not walk that path alone.

This is the hour of loss, this is the painful moment of those left behind. We all know that moment. Next comes the remembering and the healing process begins. Then comes the realization that in his few years Mark drew from us the mighty and unencumbered power of love. He moved us all in his quiet way. The cold of winter is just a breath away, the community's love for a boy and his family will not change with the seasons.

While Swansea laments the loss not just of one of its young and beautiful children, there are those who have drawn strength from the tragedy. Mark's schoolmates have grown wise beyond their tender years. They refused to abandon the friend they loved so much. They held true and close all during the months Mark appeared to be doing well, only to fade, rebound and fade again.

These wonderful children have taught us all a lesson. They refused to allow fear to dominate their lives. They looked at their classmate's health problem and did not run and did not hide. These children of Swansea refused to let the darkness obliterate the sunlight that was Mark.

No school can teach children what Mark's classmates learned about the human experience, about life and, sadly enough, death. Mark is no longer with them physically, but his spirit will always be a force in the lives of these Swansea young people. For all of us, we can only hope that the legacy of our existence is that it impacts positively on the lives of others. Mark, in his too few years, did that more than most of us. Mark thrived in school, he loved science as he loved life. He was the pride of his parents and grandparents, his Little League coaches and his neighborhood. Death may have stolen a boy from our midst, but it did not take away Mark's glowing beacon of light that will shine on us and guide us through the stormy waters of life.

A couple of weeks ago, I received a call from the news department at Columbia Broadcasting System. The Swansea story, a town that refused to reject one of its own, is of national interest. They wanted information about Mark so I referred the caller to the boy's doctor at Rhode Island Hospital.

The CBS news department was following up on a newspaper account that appeared in the nationally distributed *Christian Science Monitor*. A professor from California researched and wrote the piece. He phoned me this past summer and wanted a sense of how and why the community reacted with such compassion when in places such as New York and Kokomo, Ind., there were public protests calling for the barring of AIDS victims from schools.

I told him that in my own opinion Swansea may just be a better place with enlightened people. I also said that School Supt. John McCarthy and his staff defused the fears of many town residents by bringing forward public health experts. Swansea—from that night more than a year ago when hundreds of townspeople gathered in the high school auditorium—will remain a place where people reasoned together and rallied behind an ailing boy and his right to attend school.

The fears expressed that night just over a year ago were genuine. The questions were many. Questions were met with answers. Hysteria was not allowed to take over during that meeting. I watched as Jack McCarthy told the audience of his decision to allow Mark into school. I admired his courage, for here in our midst was a shepherd who could have easily abandoned one member of his flock but refused to do so.

There was no panic in Swansea thanks to Jack McCarthy and his colleagues but mostly because of the young and wise children of the town—a town that has passed the test of adversity and has shown to the world the depth and quality of the human spirit.

Mark touched us all. Though I never met him, I feel his presence everywhere in the town that I call home. I see Mark in the children carrying their books and boarding school buses. In our age, we gather up these experiences and store them.

Mark is like some shooting star that pierces the black of night. It catches our eye and we hold our breath in wonder. In the wake of the sighting, we await the next vision in anticipation that it will lift our souls from these earthly bonds.

In the struggle of life and death, Mark has ascended to a higher plane. The tragedy of a hemophiliac contracting AIDS through a blood transfusion has become more than the struggle of a boy and his family to deal with the personal devastation with dignity and courage. It challenged a town and an area. Town officials and citizens were tested and like few places on this good earth, they rose to the challenge and gave meaning to such words as COURAGE, COMPASSION, LEADERSHIP, FELLOWSHIP, ENLIGHTENMENT. The standards were set by a school administration but could not have been enforced except for the wonderful young people of a town where social values still mean something. Those who do not live in Swansea have benefitted by example.

In a nearby town, school officials have determined that no AIDS victim will be allowed to attend class. That is in direct violation of the state law. But beyond that, maybe the administrators could learn from Mark's classmates.

Mark was not rejected, he was embraced. No one grew ill, just better. The night holds many fears that can be erased by the dawn's early light. Mark's passage through that night has given our area a dawn bright and beautiful. Now he leaves us, but he leaves us all better for his presence.

Sadness is a heavy weight that we must carry from time to time. Mark's joy to be alive and to be part of us all will lift that burden from our shoulders. As the trees grow barren in the autumn of the year, we are sustained by the knowledge that spring will soon return and the world will come alive again.

In our time, few things will impact on so many as this one boy's struggle with a disease and one town's absolute refusal to reject a child. Mark's fate is not as tragic if his legacy is the elevation of human kindness and understanding. Rest now, Mark, your trials are over. Rise up, spirit of goodness, you were true to the end.

———————

The November issue of the Case Junior High newspaper also had some comments about Mark. Maria Resendes said, "We remember Mark, a legend in his own time. Mark had many friends that he didn't even know he had. Mark and I were very close. Knowing Mark the way I did, I can honestly say that Mark was one of the best kids that I know. It was a sad death, not only for his family, but also for his friends. People from hundreds of miles away came to see Mark. Mark was filled with spunk. He had high hopes. We, the kids at the junior high, and the freshmen at the high school, know how much Mark meant to us. We put up a big fight to let Mark attend school at the junior high. I personally feel that letting Mark attend school was the best idea. Mark was an inspiration for many kids. He taught kids that life is good and taught them not to mistreat it. Mark was never down. We will all miss Mark; we won't forget him."

———————

When I think back to the week that Mark died, I am amazed that I survived; that I didn't end up in a mental hospital. It was a crushing blow! Sons are supposed to bury fathers; fathers are not supposed to bury sons! Sons are supposed to grow up and marry some nice girl and give you grandchildren. I was walking around, going through the motions of life, but I was in shock! I was eating too much, I couldn't sleep and I was totally depressed. Only a parent who has lost a child can really understand the terrible sense of loss that eats away at your very soul.

Relatives and friends really helped. We had company at our house every day and night for months. I guess everyone grieves differently. In my case, I wanted to talk about Mark and I still do. I felt hurt when some friends didn't mention him when they saw us. I know that they probably felt awkward, but it hurt. I just lost my son! Who cares about the weather, my job, or sports?

I was very angry at God. I had prayed so hard and He hadn't answered my prayers. St. Jude, the saint of the impossible, hadn't come through for me. Neither had all the other saints to whom I had prayed so hard. I had devoted my life to teaching in a Catholic school and felt like quitting. I had promised Dale that Mark would be all right because I had really believed it.

Dale wanted to talk about Mark, too. But Scott did not want to at all. He wanted to go back to school the day after the funeral. I know he felt terrible, too, but he kept most of his emotions to himself. He felt very angry, too. He missed his brother very much. Scott and Mark were so close. They always played together. They had the same illness and understood the pain involved with hemophilia. Once in a while he would let his feelings slip out. He told us, "When I get married, I'm going to have three children, in case one dies." Scott was now an only child.

The newspaper was very painful to read. It seemed like every single day there would be an article about AIDS. Every newscast on TV also seemed to mention it.

I kept thinking, what is Mark doing now? Were our relatives who passed away taking care of him? Could he see what was going on down here on earth? I should have been there to greet him when he died. How did he feel now? Did he miss us, or was he too busy enjoying everlasting happiness? Why did he have to suffer so much and die so young? What is heaven really like?

I really began to think about God again. Maybe it was a blessing that God allowed Mark to die. Did I really want Mark to suffer anymore? No, but I did want him to get better and stay better. I expected him to beat the AIDS virus. I expected him to be cured.

I really loved Mark so much. But God is called all-loving. If my love for Mark was so great, then God's love must be infinitely greater for Mark. God must have wanted Mark very much. He must have been very special to Him. I always believed that life was a test and it was our goal to use the gifts that God had given to us to be the best that we could be. I stressed this with Mark and Scott and all my students at St. John's. Mark certainly tried his best. I knew he had to be in heaven because if he wasn't, nobody else would make it there. Not that he was perfect, but he was just a good kid.

My thoughts of quitting school vanished. Mark's philosophy—"A winner never quits and a quitter never wins"—kept popping into my mind. That's not what Mark would want me to do. He was all right, he had given me a sign through the video game.

A little black kitten showed up at our sliding glass door in the kitchen. He looked exactly like Mark's cat Tiny. We would open the door, but the kitten was too afraid to come in. Scott fed him and cared for him and eventually the kitten came in. Scott named him "Chicken." Mark had loved cats. Could this be another sign?

I began reading the New Testament again. I wanted to know every little thing that Jesus had said about heaven. I read some pages every night until I finished the entire book. Then I read every book I could find about death. I read books like *When Bad Things Happen to Good People* by Harold S. Kushner and *Life After Life* and *Reflections On Life After Life* by Raymond A. Moody, Jr., M.D. I read all of Edgar Cayce's books and Ruth Montgomery's books. I even wrote to Mrs. Montgomery and she responded. I read and read and read. Some of the books seemed really weird, while others gave me new insights into the afterlife and interested me.

Then finally I realized that death was just a natural part of living. It was probably just as easy as falling to sleep at night. Death would happen to every one of us some day. Everyone who was at Mark's funeral would some day face the same thing that Mark did. His time just came sooner. His worries were over. He didn't have to get up early for school anymore. He didn't have to worry about quizzes and tests. He didn't have to worry about a thing. God would take care of Mark. Mark would take care of us. Mark was a new saint.

I decided that it would be best for me to get right back to school as soon as possible. I called Sister Martha and told her that I would be back on Monday. I asked Dale to come with me. I didn't want her to be home alone all day. She agreed to volunteer her time. Dale was a big help to everyone at St. John's. The kids all loved her. She ran off papers for the teachers, helped correct papers, worked with small reading groups, helped in the cafeteria, took recess and yard duty, worked in the office, helped Sister Martha, and ran errands.

But every day on the way home she would cry. Seeing all those healthy kids hurt. She missed Mark so much. We comforted each other. I was happy that I had company—it was a 30-minute ride home. Each afternoon we would visit Mark's grave. We still visit the cemetery every day. We picked out a headstone with a rose, Mark's favorite flower, on it. Later someone gave me a card about roses. It said that the rose stood for short life, martyrdom, and love. It certainly was a good symbol for Mark. The headstone also had a brick wall in one corner. The brick wall reminded us of school. Mark had loved school so much that we thought the stone would be very appropriate. The stone was put in the center of the four-grave plot we purchased. We also had a flat stone put down at the exact spot of Mark's grave. All we wanted on this was "MARK." Dale spent hours and hours making floral decorations for the cemetery. She picked out a theme each month and it gave her a lot of pleasure to have his site looking so nice.

Mark was not going to be forgotten. The Friends of Mark helped pay for the funeral expenses. We did not have very much insurance on the boys because they were hemophiliacs and no company wanted to insure them. All the remaining money in the Friends of Mark account was put into the newly-formed scholarship fund.

The girls on the Case High volleyball team had a game the night of Mark's funeral. They had attended the funeral as a team that morning. They wore black ribbons on their shoulders in his memory and dedicated the game to Mark. Case won.

The St. Dominic's Confirmation Class had a raffle to raise money for the scholarship. Over $600 was raised.

The end-of-the-year reports in the local newspapers all had articles about Swansea and how it was a "caring community."

Mark's freshman class had a jewelry sale in the fall to raise money for dues and activities. Mark had even sold items himself back in late September. He had always enjoyed going house-to-house selling things for school. When the class raised $1,600, they decided to give $1,000 of it to Mark's scholarship fund.

Denny Moglia and Johnny Shaeffer, family friends, ran the Mark G. Hoyle Memorial Golf Tournament at a local golf club to raise money for the scholarship.

The annual Fay Chretian basketball game between the Case High School faculty and Case Junior High School faculty was played for Mark's scholarship. The late Fay Chretian was a cheerleader from the Class of 1962. The Chretian Committee wanted to help get Mark's scholarship going. They raised $1,097.

The Case High School Theater Company dedicated their play *Nicholas Nickleby* to Mark. The play, written by Charles Dickens, is about a boy thrown into a world for which he is not prepared. But through courage, Nicholas is able to triumph over evil through good.

In the Case program, this was said about Mark: "A young man of our community, like Nicholas, was thrust into a world that was not kind to him but he did not succumb to its hurts and insults. Instead, he stood up to all that was handed to him with a strength and valor that will serve as a constant symbol to us all! We therefore dedicate our production of *Nicholas Nickleby* to the memory of Mark Hoyle."

In March, *The Somerset Spectator* did an article about town reports for the year. Barbara Davies wrote about AIDS and how "everyone had the opportunity of seeing courage in action as the student continued his schooling." The article went on to say that Mr. McCarthy had to report that the child had died in October. Barbara Davies continued, "Mark Hoyle's contribution to all of us is the realization each has absorbed from his manner of living. Like any thought sent out into our world, the impact on each life will expand and continue, and the impact on our community will continue to be realized. The fact that Swansea and the persons most closely involved have been nationally recognized through this experience is only the visible result."

At the end of the month my family gave out the first annual Mark Hoyle Memorial Science Award. It was a plaque and a $50 savings bond. It was my brother Jeff's idea and everyone chipped in. He presented it to Anne Giovanni of Taunton Catholic Middle School. We all had gone to judge the project that we thought best met the criteria.

During the winter the Community Achievement and Scholastic Excellence Committee named Mark as an inductee of the CASE Award. "It is strongly felt that Mark's personal courage and his ability to bring a community together to support one young man's cause in a very controversial issue exemplifies the essence of the CASE Award," said the newspaper account in the *Cardinal*, the high school newspaper.

Scott continued to have bleeds and need treatment. He had nine treatments in October of '86, nine in November, 15 in December, and 25 in January. Most of the bleeds involved his left knee. The doctors decided that a knee operation would be the best thing to do for Scott. We had to go back to Rhode Island Hospital in February of '87. It was very painful for all of us. Scott ended up in one of the same rooms that his brother had been in on Potter I. Pam Cote, Marianne Carlucci, and all Mark's other nurses became Scott's nurses. Dr. E. Lowe performed the arthroscopy. It was a great success. Dr. Smith, Nancy Keyes, and Debbie DeMaio gave us excellent support (as usual). Our families also came up to visit Scott often. We stayed with him just like we had done with Mark. Later Scott had to receive many months of prophylactic treatment and do daily therapy. Sue Cotta, who had worked on Mark, came to our house weekly to help Scott do his therapy. The knee did improve, but not quickly enough to let him play Little League baseball.

Parents and students at my school started a Mark Hoyle Memorial Library Fund. Many books continue to be purchased in his memory through the generosity of the St. John community. Dale and I continue to send personal thank you notes to all who contribute to this as well as the scholarship fund.

In April, the Swansea Little League dedicated their program to the memory of Mark and two others who had passed away since the league ended in the fall. Scott was called upon to throw out the first pitch to open the season. He pitched a perfect strike to the Police Chief Ralph Lepore, Jr. He swung and missed. It is tradition that the ball has to be hit, so Scott threw another perfect pitch. This time the chief hit a ground ball to the shortstop side of the field.

A story about Mark appeared on WCVB, Channel 5, in Boston on their "Chronicle" show. The television crew came down from Boston to St. John's because we were doing AIDS education programs with the students and we were a parochial school. They showed scenes of me teaching my class. They also showed Franny Powers teaching her class. They interviewed Sister Martha and me. They used some of our home video tapes of Mark, too. The story was well done.

In May *Parenting* magazine had a feature story about Mark written by Jacques Leslie. He had come from California to interview us shortly after Mark died. It had been very difficult at the time, but the results were well worth it. Mark had always wanted to be famous and now I wanted him to get his wish. *A Tale of Two Cities* compared the way Swansea handled Mark's case with the way Atascadero, California, handled a case in their town.

David Kirp, our friend from San Francisco, is also writing about Mark in a chapter in his book which is entitled, *Suffer the Children.*

MTA Today, a magazine put out by the Massachusetts Teachers Association, also had a May issue featuring a story about Mark. Andy Linebaugh wrote the touching article. He said that, "Mark Hoyle and Jack McCarthy had something in common — courage!"

Besides having his picture in *Parenting* and *MTA Today,* the *Boston Globe* did a special memorial to AIDS victims who had died. Mark was chosen as one of the 12 to have their pictures featured. This was May 17, 1987.

On May 28, Dale and I attended Class Night Exercises at Case High School. I was called up to the stage to hand out the first Mark Gardiner Hoyle Memorial Scholarship. Valedictorian Lisa Romanovich was the choice of the scholarship committee. She received $1,000.

WPRI-TV, Channel 12, produced a special called, "Living With AIDS." One night they had a segment on Mark. Greta Kreuz interviewed me at our home and the cameras filmed Dale, Scott, the dog, and me. (Webster was our new dog that we had bought for Scott at Easter. He was half cocker spaniel and half poodle—a cockapoo.) Channel 12 also used footage from the home videos that we took of Mark. Later in July, they did another AIDS special and used additional footage of Mark.

The annual town report in Swansea, which is like a book, had a large picture of Mark on their first page. Mark was mentioned in the superintendent's report and the Case Junior High School report. The latter told how, "This year's drama production was *Annie*. Not only was this play an outstanding performance, but the song "Tomorrow," an integral part of the play, was sung at the funeral of Mark Hoyle and will long remain in the memory of those associated with the school."

The Case Junior High Yearbook was dedicated to Mark. Under his picture they had, "He who influences the thought of his time influences the thought of all the times that follow. His quiet courage was an inspiration to us all. His legacy is that by his example he made us better people."

St. John the Evangelist School also dedicated their yearbook to Mark. They said that Mark "was and always will be an inspiration to us all. Mark taught us all a very important lesson, one that will guide us through our lives. He taught us to live as full a life as possible and to make the best out of what seems to be the worst. Mark is our hero and we'll never forget him." They also had a poem written by Kristone which they said best described Mark's motto in life.

When my class graduated in June, Melissa Menard, a class officer, said a few words about Mark and then presented me with a nice plaque. "In loving memory of Mark Gardiner Hoyle, August 2, 1972–October 26, 1986, dedicated from Class of '87." It also had Mark's saying, "A winner never quits, a quitter never wins. It's never too late to rally," along with two crossed baseball bats and a baseball. My generous class also donated $100 to Mark's scholarship fund and $90 to Mark's Memorial Library Fund.

In June, the Case Junior High administration, faculty, and workers bought an evergreen tree and planted it outside the art room in Mark's memory. A cement plaque, near the foot of the tree, is shaped like a home plate with Mark's name as well as a bat and ball engraved on it.

There was a national all-night television special on about

AIDS in July. The *Chronicle* footage about Mark and St. John's was seen all over the country. Channel 12-WPRI-TV, broke into the program with their own half-hour special which included the footage they shot about Mark. This was just shown locally, however.

During Mark's last hospital stay, my mother was sitting up with him one night and she wrote a poem, which she entitled "My Prayer to God." In one stanza she wrote, "And I want him to say 'Hi Nan' to me." On July 7, 1987, almost nine months after his death, she had an answer to that poem.

On that hot, sunny July day, my parents went to Mt. Hope Cemetery to visit Mark's grave as they did every other day. They got out of their car and prayed. My father then got back into the car since he has emphysema and the heat was bothering him. My mother remained to pray some more and to think about Mark. All of a sudden my mother heard a voice say loud and clearly, "Hi Nan!" It startled her. She turned around quickly to see if Scott had come by with me since we often met there. She thought it had been Scott's voice she heard. But when she turned to look, no one was around but my father who was sitting in the car with the air conditioner on and the windows shut.

My mother started to cry. It had to be Mark's voice that she had heard. He always called her "Nan" instead of Nana. She quickly went to see if my father had heard anything, but he hadn't. It was a message meant only for her ears.

The August 10, 1987, edition of *Newsweek* featured "The Face of AIDS—One Year in the Epidemic." Mark's picture was one of the 24 shown on the cover. Inside, his picture appeared with others who had passed away in October of 1986. Under his picture it said, "Mark Hoyle, 14, Swansea, Mass. An honor student, star athlete—and hemophiliac."

Dan Fagan, a newspaper staff writer from the *Saratoga Herald-Tribune*, called me for an interview about Mark in August. He later sent me a copy of his August 16 story. It dealt with Swansea, Atascadero, and Arcadia, Florida. As in the *Parenting* article, Swansea set the example.

On the 23rd of August, we were embarrassed to find our pictures on the front page of the Sunday *Fall River Herald-News*. I had agreed to talk to Fred Rhines about the book I was writing. But we never expected the picture and article to be right there on the front page. Dale and I were both in very sad moods that day and looked terrible, but Scott looked fine. The part I will always remember about the article is the last two paragraphs because they made me sad. "There are memories," it said, "in the backyard, where a great, old maple tree stands near the patio.

"A well-constructed treehouse, painted steel gray and complete with ladder for entry, stands with its door ajar in that old tree—waiting for a smiling young boy who never will return."

In August, the Swansea Little League held their first annual Mark G. Hoyle Memorial Tournament for 9- and 10- year-olds. We all went down to the opening ceremonies and Scott threw out the first ball. Later, all the coaches and players on the Swansea All-Star team signed the ball. Mark and Scott had both played in the 9- and 10-year-old tourney during their Little League years. Now it would be named for Mark. I'm sure he would be proud. Maplewood of Fall River won the hard-fought tournament. We attended many of the games and were present to hand out the trophies. We also were given a gift by the Swansea Little League. It was a nice plaque which said, "In Memory of Mark Hoyle—1st Annual Memorial Tournament Swansea Little League 1987."

"Arcadia, Florida, could have taken a lesson from Swansea" was the September 1 headline in Mark Patinkin's column. It was the fourth time that he had devoted a column to Mark and Swansea. Mark Patinkin had called me and written about the two different ways that the towns had handled the AIDS situation.

The September 7 issue of *Newsweek* also mentioned Mark on page 53. It talked about how "Americans were capable of reacting with considerable warmth and courage when confronted with the AIDS-in-school dilemma."

Many articles about Mark appeared in other newspapers, magazines, and even school weeklies across the country. But the main point, as Mr. Devine said so well in a "Guest Spot" in *The Spectator*: " . . . we must not forget what happened in one small Massachusetts town. A town in which decent people were able to overcome fear and emotion. A town in which compassion and understanding prevailed. A town whose people can remember with pride that they cared. When Mark Hoyle died last year, our whole community shared in the loss. His parents' grief became our grief. We as a community could take comfort in the knowledge that the quality of Mark's life was as good as possible. His final year was one of hope and happiness. Mark loved his family and his friends and his school and community; and they loved him."

A chicken barbecue was held in September to raise money for the scholarship. My brother-in-law, Ken Gardiner, ran it and it raised over $1,700. The Friends of Mark held a Scholarship Dance in October which also added to the scholarship funds.

Also in October, my family was invited to attend the Maplewood Little League banquet. We helped distribute trophies to the All-Stars who had won Mark's first tournament. Tony Rocha, the president of the League, then gave us a beautiful plaque which said, "Presented to the Hoyle Family from the Winners of the First Annual Mark Hoyle Memorial Tournament Maplewood 9–10 All Stars 1987." The top half of the plaque had a team picture of the champs.

The Case Junior High Parent-Teacher Organization has donated science books to the Media Center in memory of Mark. They also have made a collage of photos, yearbook dedications, and personal items of Mark for display.

So many kind gestures have been made in memoriam of Mark—each one gives us continued comfort and strength. And we are continually heartened that the tributes haven't stopped. For instance, Kathleen Ryan, one of Mark's tutors, drew a beautiful, lifelike portrait of Mark and the Friends of Mark will be presenting it to Case High School. To add to Mark's scholarship fund, the Somerset Runners Club and Excellent Pizza of Somerset, Massachusetts, have announced a three-mile race with all proceeds to go to the scholarship fund. Mark, you must be smiling.

Of course, the media also continues to call upon our experiences in its efforts to inform the public about AIDS. Century III Teleproductions of Boston contacted us about incorporating

Mark's story into a television special. The City of New York Commission on Human Rights also contacted us about a future television special on AIDS. They, too, want to include Mark's story.

In the fall, WLNE, Channel 6, interviewed me at our home. They were so impressed with the Sports Room that we taped the interview there. Right after Mark had died, we thought it best to take down his room and, besides, Scott wanted the larger bedroom. Before dismantling the room, I videotaped it as Mark had designed it so that we would have a permanent record.

We set Scott up with a new waterbed, wallpaper, and rug. We made Scott's old room into a Sports Room in Mark's memory. On one wall we have a giant poster of both Mark and Scott at Fenway Park. We have surrounded it with autographed baseball cards that fill the entire wall. Another wall is for Mark's autographed pictures of celebrities. On the third wall are Little League pictures of the boys, along with other sports memorabilia. The final wall has a shelf unit filled with baseball cards. I have spent many hours writing this book in that Sports Room.

The memory of Mark and his courage will live on in my heart forever. I am very proud of the way my son handled all the challenges that he faced. I am also very proud of Swansea, our hometown.

Until we meet again, Mark, I love you and pray that God takes great care of you for me. I'll miss you always. Love, Dad.
12/18/87